There is an implicit contract ↑
Certain expectations are in plac
*conventionally considered the natural order of things. With a clear eye—and with
no emotional manipulation whatsoever—Robert Waxler tells us what happens
when that contract goes awry. This is a very important story, beautifully told. The
story of Robert, Linda and Jeremy—with Jonathan hovering close by—reminds
us that a parent's love for a child truly knows no bounds.*

– Elizabeth Mehren, Professor of Journalism, Boston University, author of *Born Too Soon*

*A literature professor and writer, Bob Waxler offers here a compelling story that
reads at times like a medical thriller, at times like a philosophic meditation, and at
times like a family tale of fear and hope. I greatly admire his son Jeremy's courage
to face such difficult odds after his sudden spinal trauma, and I am inspired by
the well-trained physicians who helped make his recovery possible. Perhaps most,
though, I am moved by the way the poetry throughout the story allows us to glimpse
how close to a miracle this whole experience really is.*

Dr. Al Rabson, Deputy Director National Cancer Institute, National Institute of Health

*Robert Waxler's book provides a poignant and troubling look at a family struggling
courageously in the face of a harrowing crisis. What happens when a son is stricken
with a mysterious and potentially fatal disease? Why does this happen and how does
one—how can one—understand this? What can be done when so much feels out of
control? Who should make which decisions? These and other issues are confronted
in Mr. Waxler's unsettling, absorbing and compelling narrative, which speaks to the
heart as well as the mind.*

Dr. Francis Haines, Assistant Professor of Psychiatry, Brown University

*As someone with cerebral palsy who also works in the disability field, I am acutely
aware of the unique challenges that disability can bring to individuals and their
families. Professor Waxler's book combines humor, emotion and personal reflection
to create a refreshingly honest and accurate look at the highs and lows involved
for the entire family after his son Jeremy's illness.* Courage to Walk *is a winner!*

Patrick Gleason, Staff Writer Eunice Kennedy Shriver Center Spotlight Newsletter

*When Bob Waxler's son Jeremy fell, his parents' lives took a sharp turn neither
one would have chosen. In this uncharted territory, desperate for his son's return to
health, Bob Waxler teetered between the abysses of immersion and loss. To find his
path, he turned to literature, or more accurately, he turned his life into literature. By
offering us the story of the those dark days, Waxler sheds light on the love between
a father and his son and on the relationship between life and literature.*

Jerry Waxler, M.S., author, lecturer, and therapist

Courage to Walk

Text © 2010 Robert Waxler

All rights reserved.
© Spinner Publications, Inc.
New Bedford, Massachusetts 02740
Printed in the United States of America

Library of Congress Cataloging-in-Publication Data

Waxler, Robert P., 1944-
 Courage to walk / Robert Waxler.
    p. cm.
 ISBN 978-0-932027-64-1 (alk. paper)
 1. Waxler, Jeremy, 1974—Health. 2. Paraplegics—United States—Biography. 3. Spinal cord—Diseases—Patients—United States—Biography. 4. Fathers and sons. 5. Paraplegics—Rehabilitation.
 I. Title.
 RC406.P3W39 2010
 617.4'82—dc22
                                          2010001454

Courage to Walk

Robert Waxler

Spinner Publications, Inc.
New Bedford, Massachusetts

To Jeremy and Linda

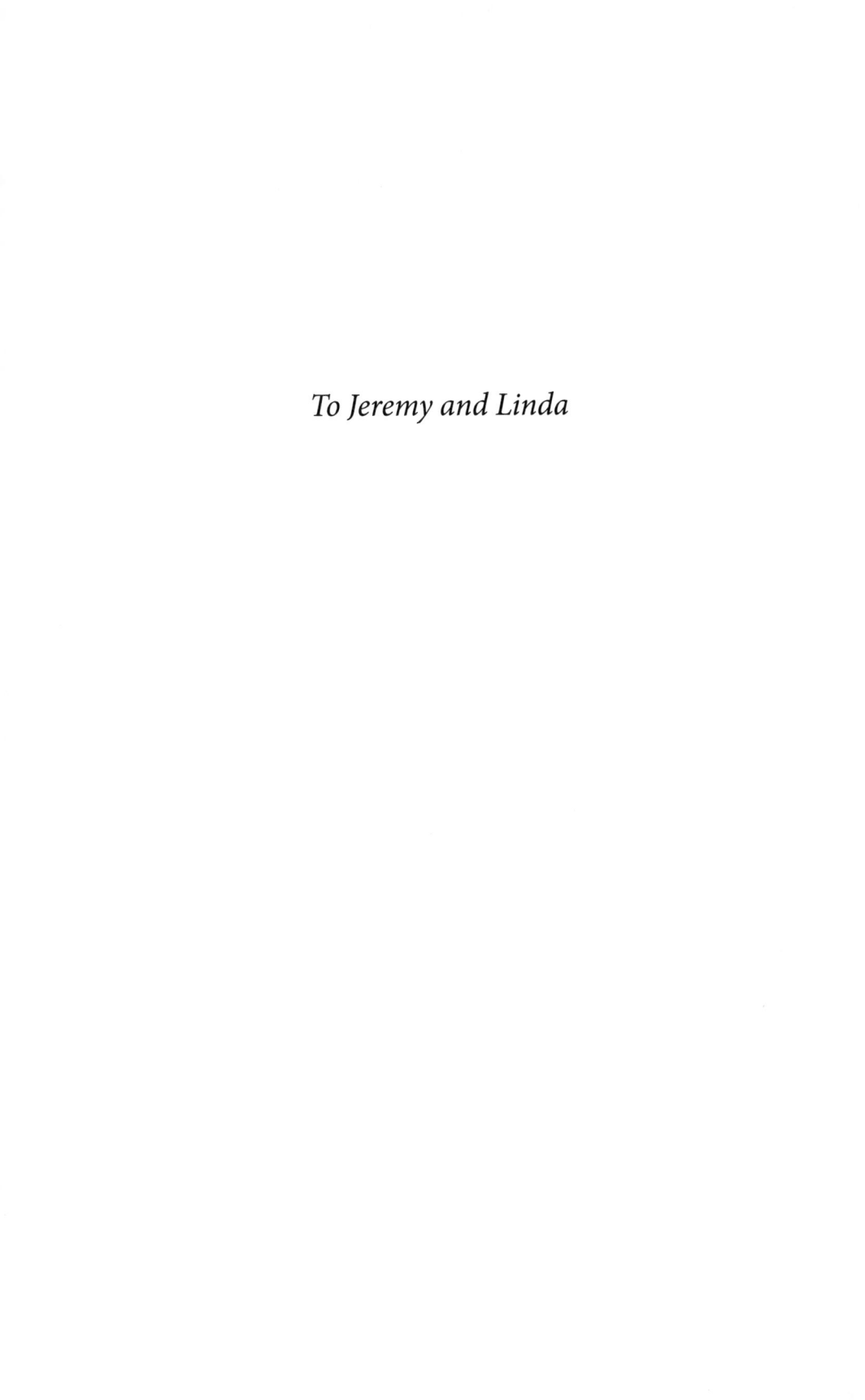

Acknowledgments

There are always wonderful people to thank for making a book possible. *Courage to Walk* is no exception.

I especially want to thank Jeremy and Linda. Jeremy, your courage throughout this difficult journey was inspirational, and I know readers, each step of the way, will find such courage uplifting. Linda, your optimism in the midst of such turmoil will always stand as a valuable lesson for all of us. I love you both with all my heart, and I dedicate this book to you.

Howard Senzel, Carl Schinasi, Elizabeth Mehren, Jerry Waxler and Jim Nee—thank you so much for your willingness to read and reread my early drafts. From the beginning, your critical and sensitive comments kept me alert and helped me shape the story as it developed.

I am also grateful to Elissa Ely, Francis Haines, Jane Lindenbaum, Kate and Joe Madigan, Donna and Dennis Manna, Bradie Metheny, Susan Newman and Mickey Lowenstein, Al Rabson, Adrienne and Joel Rosenblatt, Evie and David Sarles and Helen Waxler. Your advice and encouragement made more of a difference than you might imagine.

And, of course, thank you to all the people at Spinner Publications: Joe Thomas, whose support is always important to me, and Marsha McCabe, Heather Haggerty, Jay Avila and Claire Nemes, for their quality work.

The Hospital

The table is blue pearl granite, and I have a sonnet by Rilke, printed out from my iMac, lying on that hard stone, waiting patiently to be read. I look out across my study to the crafted shelves lining three walls, shelves overflowing with books and journals. I carefully fasten my glasses—wire-rimmed and professorial—around my ears and look down:

> *Be ahead of all parting, as though it already were*
> *Behind you, like the winter that has just gone by.*
> *For among these winters there is one so endlessly winter*
> *That only by wintering through it will your heart survive.*

Perhaps I can discuss this poem with my literature class this fall, I think, wondering where the time has gone, contemplating the possibility of retirement from the university in a year or two. It is easy to think this way in the midst of summer, the July breeze gently circling through the window, caressing the poem, lifting it slightly from the hard granite. On this warm Sunday evening, shadows of dusk dart across the lawn beneath my window, birds sing in the trees. It's the closing of a glorious day of celebration, a day sparkling with birthday candles and two cakes, one for our son Jeremy at thirty-three, one for my elderly mother at ninety.

How many days can be like this in a lifetime, I wonder, as I leave my study and go outdoors to ramble barefoot through the green grass. It is as if I am walking through a poem, Mary Oliver's "The Summer Day."

"Who made the world?" the poet asks, while I wander inside her creation—a grasshopper flinging herself out of the green grass, snapping her wings open and then floating away.

The light dims, the shadows dance across the lawn, the dusk shapes and reshapes flickering patterns on the grass, and I am wrapped again in the poet's words:

> *Doesn't everything die at last, and too soon?*
> *Tell me, what is it you plan to do*
> *With your one wild and precious life?*

Rilke and Oliver. Perhaps I can use both poems in my class this fall, the same effect achieved by such profoundly different voices. It is all an endless surprise, I think, as the moon brightens in the night sky, just a sliver of pale fire shining through the dark clouds.

One never knows for sure.

∽

Just eight years ago, they posted the results of Jeremy's law boards on the Internet.

Working for the Secretary of State, fresh out of law school, Jeremy glanced through his office window out to the Boston Harbor that day. The bright sun glistened on the blue water, boats bobbed at their moorings. But he was not really interested in that view; for him, that perspective was merely a temporary distraction, a fleeting glimpse through glass at a distance. Jeremy focused instead on the electronic images flickering on the computer screen right in front of him. He was searching for something that he could hold onto, something that might guarantee him purpose and direction.

Jeremy must have stared at that computer for several hours, checking and rechecking. Then, like magic, a list popped up very late in the afternoon. Countless names in alphabetical order. The list seemed to materialize from nowhere, now suddenly there on the screen, ready to be read.

Jeremy sat straight up. His thick back, draped in a blue suit, pressed against the chair; he bent forward, his red tie loosely hanging from his neck. He scrolled down the long list of names, rapidly working his way through the alphabet. He was holding his breath the whole time, his skin warm with beads of sweat. Finally, he arrived at the *Ws*. He paused at the keyboard, and then started again, cautiously reading each name on the electronic screen, one at a time, until he spotted the one name, the only one, he had been searching for. He read the name to himself in a whisper: "Waxler, Jeremy R."

The telephone rang off the hook in my office in the English department. "Dad, I'm a lawyer," he shouted, his voice filled with the wonder of someone who had just sauntered into a new world. His eyes peered through the glass window in his office; they darted across the Boston Harbor. They scanned the ocean, following the curve of time far out to the distant horizon.

> *Tell me, what is it you plan to do*
> *With your one wild and precious life?*

∼

Adult children are always still your children, no matter how old they are. You stay attached to them forever. Their joy is your joy; their terror your terror. That bond, established at birth, stretches through a lifetime; it continues beyond the grave. That bond is timeless, everlasting.

The evening after that enchanted birthday party at our house, Jeremy finishes up at his law office on Sixth Street in New Bedford. He stacks his files neatly on his desk, and we drive to the Venus de Milo restaurant in Swansea. Just the three of us. Linda, Jeremy and I. It is Monday, July 16, the official date of his birth. We celebrate his birthday like this each year: "Overstuffed lobsters at the Venus de Milo," we shout, and then we're off, up the old Route 6, eager to gather around the restaurant table, the three of us laughing and talking and cracking the big red lobster claws. Jeremy could be thirteen or twenty-three or thirty-three, I think to myself at that table. He will always be our son, and I will always be his father, Linda his mother, no matter how old we all get. I am always glad to be with him and Linda on such nights, toasting to his future, participating in these wide-grin rituals we reenact together as a tightly knit family each and every year.

To me, the young lawyer, Jeremy, is the same son who stood, proud and erect, illuminating a small stage at the local elementary school one night long ago. His feet moved back and forth then, strong legs shuffling about on that fragile platform. Like the other students, he was restless that starry night, waiting for the school superintendent to announce the next word through the screeching microphone, while the crowd remained hushed on the edge of their seats in the old auditorium.

Jeremy listened intently, reflecting on each word presented to him, until, one by one, his classmates were eliminated, leaving him, finally, standing with one other young student on that big wooden stage. He was only in the fifth grade then, anxious yet confident.

The superintendent leaned into the microphone, peering across the stage at the girl who had just moved forward to take her turn. "The word is *knives*," he bellowed. "Can you please use it in a sentence?" the young girl squirmed in reply, twisting her hair with her fingers.

The superintendent smiled as he slowly formed the sentence: "The mother set the knives on the table for supper." The girl hesitated, shuffled about, and then finally spelled the word out: K-N-I-F-E-S.

We heard the groan and felt the disappointment in the humid air as she retreated back to her spot on the stage, and Jeremy stepped up to give it his try.

The superintendent leaned in again: "The word is *scissors*," he said.

Standing straight, Jeremy started right in, not letting anyone take a breath: S-C-I-S-S-O-R-S. The auditorium erupted with applause this time. Jeremy had won the city-wide spelling bee! We were all in an uproar.

It was a moon-drenched night, as I recall. The golden trophy was almost as big as he was. Jeremy proudly carried it from the car into the house that evening. He was beaming. The champion, he glowed for a week from ear to ear. We all did.

I watch him now dig into his lobster, a bright smile across his face. "Jeremy, do you remember when we went down to Florida that December a few years ago?" We had headed south to see the bureaucrats trying to clarify the presidential election: Bush vs. Gore. "Remember, we sat in the visitor's gallery watching them check each ballot?"

"Yes, I remember, Dad," Jeremy says, laughing and taking a sip of beer from his glass. "Those guys were ridiculous. Remember how they raised each ballot to the light and looked up at those hanging chads? They were pretending to read the voter's intention. I couldn't believe it then, and I can't believe it now."

Yes, he is the same son, the same one who was on the grammar school stage that restless evening and in the Palm Beach Court House that strange December day, the same son who has grown with us for the last thirty-three years.

"And remember what you said to the *Boston Globe* reporter when she came over to get a quote from you?" I ask him as he cracks one of his lobster claws.

"I thought I should come and see because it's history being made," he replies without hesitation.

I was proud to be there with him in Palm Beach on that weird and historic occasion, and I am proud to be sitting across the table from him tonight, celebrating his thirty-third birthday at the Venus de Milo.

∼

Two days later, Wednesday, Jeremy calls from his two-bedroom apartment located a couple of miles from our home in Dartmouth.

"My back is killing me," he tells Linda. "I can hardly get out of bed."

"Maybe you twisted it," she replies, worrying, as mothers do, about her son's pain.

"Well, maybe," he says, hesitating, assessing Linda's suggestion. "I was trying to move my bureau last night. But I didn't feel anything then."

His primary physician, Bob Sawyer, confirms on the phone what we all believe. "Ah, a little backache is nothing to be concerned about, especially with Jeremy."

The doctor would say just that, of course; I expect it. Dr. Sawyer is a compassionate and caring man, and Jeremy is strong and broad-shouldered, ordinarily brimming with robust health. Four times a week, Jeremy rides the exercise bike at the gym, pumping his legs hard, while sweat pours from his flesh. Perhaps he needs a little pain medication for his back right now, some bed rest for a few days, but he'll be fine by Saturday, we're sure. At the end of the weekend, he will be ready to return to his law office, eager to prepare for his next trial.

So we wait, Jeremy noting small signs of improvement over the next day or so, while he sits at home, following his doctor's orders. It's a torturous backache, but nothing more.

Or is it? Late Friday afternoon, Jeremy calls again. He sounds jumpy and distressed.

"I can't move my legs at all," he explains, muffled fear in his voice.

It's not what we expect. Our son is frozen in his bed. His body is not working.

∼

We planned our vacation trip six months ago: Finished with the summer session at the university, I would leave with Linda on Saturday, July 21, from Kennedy Airport in New York and fly to Madrid; then we'd board our Celebrity cruise ship on Monday and travel for two weeks across the sparkling Mediterranean to Greece. That was the plan.

Linda and I assume we are still on schedule when we drive the couple of miles over to Jeremy's apartment that Friday after his call. We are thinking that everything will be all right, that this is only a backache Jeremy has now, a painful backache for certain, causing weakness in his legs no doubt, but nothing too serious, nothing that would shake you deep down through the marrow of your bones.

Jeremy lives by himself on the second floor of an extensive modern complex. His apartment houses a small kitchen and dining area near the entrance, with washer and dryer tucked away in a corner. In the living room, his couch with its faded plaid pillows, his scratched coffee table and torn easy chair, his big-screen television, all give him comfort, a sense of being home. His Red Sox poster and a brilliant watercolor painting of the local fishing pier hang on the wall; books are scattered everywhere. They, too, seem part of him. Down a short corridor, old law files sit on a chipped wooden desk in a small second bedroom; across the way, a bathroom is kept spotless for guests.

When Linda and I pull up at his apartment, we're quiet but tense. We rush up the stairs and race through the living room, saying nothing. We pause at the threshold of the master bedroom. Jeremy lies there on his side, stretched out in the middle of his large king-sized bed, helpless on the hard mattress. Wrapped tightly in bedcovers, his body seems stiff, mummified. Jeremy looks up at us, and then we seem to glide, drifting through silence across the room. At his bedside, I gently remove the pale-blue blanket so I can get a grip from underneath his body.

"We're going to try to help you stand; then we'll check all this out at the hospital. I'm sure it'll be fine," I claim.

"Okay," he replies. "But I don't think I can walk."

Linda by my side, I bend over our son, sliding my arms beneath his rigid back. Jeremy pushes and I pull, inching across the rumpled sheets. At the edge of the bed, we stop. I tighten my arms around his midsection, secure my grip. When I lift him, the weight of his tense body presses against my hands. He slips from my grasp and falls toward the floor.

For a moment, Jeremy is stuck between the bed and the wall, suspended in air; Linda and I shove the bed aside, releasing him. He's flat on the floor, pain radiating through his back.

∽

"We've got to phone for some help."

Linda dials 911 on her cell phone, and then flies down the stairs to the street to wait for the ambulance. Minutes later, two men bolt up the stairs, following her lead. They immediately raise Jeremy off the floor and cautiously place him back on the bed.

He's settled on the mattress, but these strangers seem to stare at me, their faces odd, their eyes grim. They appear as if at a distance: their voices detached, their words howling from gaping mouths. "We'll have to call for more help before we bring your son down," they say. "We don't want to hurt him."

We stand quietly gazing at each other—it seems forever. Finally, two other men rush from the walkway, their shoes thumping up the flight of stairs. As they approach, Jeremy's body, wrenched with pain, relaxes.

"All right. Let's get him into the ambulance," they shout as they catch their breath and gain focus.

The four strangers lift our son off the bed, place him on a narrow stretcher and carry him out of the bedroom through the living room and down the narrow staircase. In a burst of sunlight, they hoist the gurney high and then slide Jeremy into the back of the ambulance. Linda and I stand stunned at the curb.

The doors of the ambulance wide open, the paramedics secure the stretcher for the ten-minute ride to the hospital. Jeremy cringes, his face mirroring our concern. Then they pull away, the wagon rumbling down the street.

"How serious can a backache be, anyway?" I ask Linda, as we follow in our car, moving toward St. Luke's. She gazes straight out through the windshield and silently shakes her head, the curls in her hair swaying back and forth until we pass by the old Dartmouth Town Hall.

∼

Like a tiger bounding from our house, Jeremy burned over to that same old Town Hall fifteen years ago on a blazing morning. His legs moved with blinding speed, his bright eyes focused on some deep distance. A special day for him, he was on fire.

At that Town Hall, he raced to the clerk behind the counter. He could hardly wait. "Could you sign me up so I can vote in the next election?" he asked. "It's my eighteenth birthday today."

"Certainly, young man," she replied, laughing when she saw him standing there, so bold with anticipation: "But which form do you want? The one to become a Democrat or the one to become a Republican?"

She was struck, she told him, by his soaring desire to exercise his right to vote, by his bright presence at the Town Hall on the morning of his birthday.

"Well," Jeremy said, "I'm delighted." But he was already picking at the chipped wood in front of him, his twinkling eyes beginning to flash with mischievous delight. "I have to tell you, though, I'm not really a Democrat or a Republican," he continued with a slight curve in his voice.

The clerk seemed baffled then, puzzled by such a reply. "Not really a Democrat or a Republican?" she finally asked with a murmur. "I'm not sure I understand."

"I'd like to register as a Communist," Jeremy burst out, a big grin lighting up his face, not a trace of irony in his tone.

He wasn't exactly kidding at the Town Hall that day.

And he isn't kidding now. He's lying in the back of an ambulance. He can barely move.

∼

The emergency ward at St. Luke's is crowded, and everyone seems to be moving in slow motion. We wait in a tight cubicle with Jeremy for close to three hours, and as we do, I begin to sense that perhaps I have made a mistake.

"Can I have a glass of water?" he asks, thirsty, wincing with pain on the gurney.

"No, I'm sorry. You have to wait for the doctor to come in."

We wait, and I pace, back and forth, pent up—a frustrated bird with clipped wings desperately wanting to fly. Linda sits quietly on a metal chair, side by side with her son, saying little.

Periodically, Linda wanders, disappearing from the room. She updates our good neighbors, Dennis and Donna, who have arrived from a dinner party to comfort us. She roams the hospital grounds. On her cell phone, she talks to Cindy, our travel agent, in case we have to cancel our vacation trip. She calls her cousin, Susan, in Chicago to keep her informed.

Technicians appear in the cubicle; they need to draw blood from Jeremy's arm, they say. They fumble with the syringe and laugh out loud when they can't find a suitable vein. Then, like apparitions, they too disappear.

"Where is the ER doctor?" I want to know. It's been three hours and the battery-driven clock on the wall ticks so slowly.

An overworked doctor, Sam Shen, finally enters the cubicle to examine Jeremy. He grasps his stethoscope and listens carefully to Jeremy's heart and lungs. He probes Jeremy's rectum, he thumbs his pulse, monitors his blood pressure, looks in his eyes and up his nose. When I stare at Shen, he appears calm at the surface of his body, but out of focus. Just below the skin he seems distressed, as if there's a shimmering boundary drawn just beneath his flesh.

Dr. Shen seems ghost-like to me, as the walls of the cubicle contract, threatening suffocation. Suddenly, the doctor raises Jeremy's right leg up off the gurney and then slowly lets it go from his bony hands. Can Jeremy keep the leg suspended in the air? Linda and I watch in horror as the leg quickly drops—like a heavy sack, like dead weight pulled by gravity to the hard ground.

We shuffle about near the nurses' station, waiting to hear Dr. Shen's assessment. The emergency ward is cramped with patients; technicians push carts filled with medical supplies; attendants rapidly move through the corridors. We are all slipping deeper and deeper into the late evening, Friday night, the beginning of the weekend.

We focus on the doctor; he seems disturbed: "This could be very serious. But I can't be sure," he says.

"What are you talking about?" I ask in response.

"Well, further tests. An MRI at least. I'm particularly concerned by the rectal examination. I feel a weakness in the soft tissue."

Dr. Shen urges us to move Jeremy immediately to Beth Israel Hospital in Boston. "They can provide more expansive treatment and testing," he says. "I'll help arrange the transfer if you want. I did my residency there. It's what you should do."

Why can't we get some answers here, I want to know. Why can't they do these tests in our local hospital, make a diagnosis closer to home? But the doctor keeps pressing, his tone pulling at me—and finally, I agree. More than his authority, his insistence moves me. "It's what you should do."

Linda wipes beads of sweat from her face with a tissue, as we both struggle against what we are hearing from the doctor, and then, glancing at each other, we embrace. "We'll have to cancel the cruise," I say. "Let Cindy know. She'll take care of the details."

An orderly appears, then quickly disappears, wheeling Jeremy out of the cubicle through the busy corridors, down a ramp. Like a phantom, he places Jeremy in a waiting wagon outside, which speeds straight to the Boston hospital. We hurry to the parking lot with my brother, David, who has come to give us support.

"Let's all drive up to Boston in my car," he suggests. "It'll be easier. Calm you down."

"No, you travel with us, if you want," I respond. "Or we'll meet you there." I sense we'll need our own vehicle in Boston tonight.

∽

The road is quiet as we move up Route 140, near the Taunton mall, and then over to Route 24, speeding past the Burger King to Route 95, through Milton onto the Jamaica Way—tree-lined, the big pond on the left—headed to Beth Israel in Boston.

When I glimpse the city lights in the far sky, I wonder if the ambulance has already pulled into the dock at the emergency ward at

Beth Israel. Is Jeremy still lying on the gurney, strapped down in the back of that wagon, attendants at his side?

I'd like to be there, release him from that gurney, take him with me in flight to the sun.

> *Daedalus fashioned wings, arranged the feathers in order,*
> *Bound them with linen and wax; soon the marvel was done.*
> *Daedalus' son stood by, fooling with wax and the feathers,*
> *Happy, like any boy, all unaware of the why.*

"Follow me where I lead, as I go flying before you," I whisper to Jeremy, hoping he can hear these words from the poet Ovid.

Then he puts on his own wings, I imagine, and adjusts them carefully; as I am about to take off, I kiss him—once is hardly enough—and there are tears in his eyes.

We are airborne, on a wonderful way, and thanks to Ovid, all the fear is forgotten for a moment as we soar.

∽

Despite the late hour at the ER, Beth Israel is bustling and alert. Infectious disease experts, neurologists, surgeons, nurses are all ready to scrutinize Jeremy. They surround him, test him, work diligently to discover what invisible creature is haunting his body. I credit Dr. Shen for his foresight, applaud him for calling ahead and prepping the Boston team.

At two in the morning, I hover over Jeremy. The doctors have inserted a catheter into his body, draining three days' urine into a plastic bag. They need to relieve his aching bladder.

Gazing at my son, I wonder where I am. We've crossed into a surreal dream, a sort of scorched wilderness where Linda and I roam. We have been thrown here, into some other country, for some unknown transgression we have committed.

Linda and I have dwelt here before, with our first son, Jonathan, his death at twenty-six from the bad heroin bought on the streets of San

Francisco in 1995 still vibrating, as it always will, through the nerves of all who loved him, screaming through our dreams still, twelve years later.

We've done what we can to avoid this other territory for the last dozen years. But there it is again, this time our younger son, the young lawyer, our only living son, battered down on the hospital sheets, tired and groggy. Jeremy can't move his legs. One would think it would have been enough with Jonathan. But apparently not. We have no choice but to follow him now into this other place, blowing with the truth of a bitter wind. As Elizabeth Barr described it:

> *Winds of the desert that sweep the long plains,*
> *Sand choke the rivers and dry up the wells,*
> *Blind the thin moon on her desolate trail,*
> *Time and the wind, the wind and the sands.*
>
> *Bitter the winds are, the high winds of home,*
> *Truthful and bitter and keen as a blade,*
> *Bitter as love are the high winds of home,*
> *Truthful as hate are the high winds of home.*

To my horror, my surreal dream is no dream at all.

~

The staff at Beth Israel, attentive and hospitable, offer us a bed in a small room down the corridor to rest, if not sleep, for a few hours if we can. They are like friendly neighbors opening a tent of comfort.

"We use that room ourselves," they tell us. "You're welcome to it."

They take blood tests, a spinal tap, an MRI of Jeremy's lower back. A young intern works endlessly on a computer, researching impossibilities. "This is so weird," he keeps insisting. "I'm going to find something," he promises.

They are intense and focused, in pursuit of a secret. They desire to know: What possibly could be causing Jeremy's pain and paralysis? What strange mystery whispers through our son's limbs?

The early results stitch a small pocket of hope for us: no visible evidence of a full-blown trauma yet. My brother travels home for the night to his wife and three children. Linda leaves to lie down in the bed granted to us.

Restless, I pace up and down the hospital corridor, while an orderly takes Jeremy for a second MRI.

"This time we'll get a full picture of his entire spinal cord," they tell me.

What if they had never done that second MRI—the one that lights up the computer screen, the one that illuminates the mass and reveals the danger? An infection, spreading up and down the spinal column, the length of four vertebrae along the back, is pressing directly on the cord, closing off complex circuits throughout Jeremy's body. What if they had never done that second MRI?

"This time of night technicians in India read these computer screens," a nurse says. "Earlier it was probably people in London. We've alerted a neurosurgeon at home in Boston, part of our team. Right now he's looking closely at the digital images flickering across the electronic grid."

I am dazzled by that, dizzy in space.

∽

Our son cannot move his legs, the legs that have evoked romance over the years and endured disappointment, the legs that have carried him to love and to heartache, too.

After he graduated from Tufts University with a political science degree, he shared a studio apartment, three flights up on Beacon Street, with a young woman who had come to Boston like a gentle breeze from Ohio after college. The couple lived together for a year before they married. Like romance itself, the sunrise illuminated their horizon each morning; rainbows glittered in the far distance after the rain. Jonathan must have sent this sparkling angel to Jeremy for comfort and confidence, Linda thought at the time.

It seemed true, just as the poet Milton put it:

> *The world was all before them, where to choose*
> *Their place of rest, and Providence their guide.*
> *They, hand in hand, with wandering steps and slow,*
> *Through Eden took their solitary way.*

The first couple, strolling out, hand in hand, from Eden. That was the way I first envisioned it. An English professor, I often see the world through the incandescent lens of poetry and stories. For me that way of seeing offers hope, at times truth. Yes, they were the perfect couple, Adam and Eve, in the beginning. That's the way I imagine Jeremy telling it, a sturgeon moon shining down on him:

> *I walked to a gazebo on the Boston Common at dusk, holding hands with my fiancée. The freshly cut grass smelled sweet, like the intoxicating fragrance of perfume in the clear air. I kneeled on both knees and then pulled the diamond ring from my pocket. The stone glittered in my hand, and my cheeks burned bright red with passion, my body fiery in the radiant glow of the evening sun. Then I dared to ask her: "Will you marry me?" My legs (yes, legs so strong then) trembled, just a little, on the soft wooden floor. "Yes, Jeremy, yes. Yes, of course, I'll marry you," she replied without hesitation.*

He was like a tiger then, embracing his own vulnerability. There is great courage in that, daring to open the heart to another. Such moments illuminate the darkness, inspire hope and create beauty in the thick forests of experience.

> *Tyger Tyger burning bright*
> *In the forest of the night;*
> *What immortal hand or eye,*
> *Dare frame thy fearful symmetry?* – William Blake

And then, a few months later, the wedding ceremony outdoors at the Toledo Country Club: A river gurgling beside the smooth green lawn on that late-May weekend; a lone sailboat gliding on the glistening water, gracing the glittering sky; and the music—yes, the music soaring like a skylark's song, the notes resonating through the warm air.

Later that night, we were all in flight, the band playing Lee Ann Womack's "I Hope You Dance":

> *Promise me that you'll give faith a fighting chance*
> *And when you get the choice to sit it out or dance*
> *I hope you—dance.*

And Bob Seger's "Old Time Rock and Roll":

> *Still like that old time rock and roll*
> *That kind of music just soothes my soul*
> *I reminisce about the days of old*
> *With that old time rock and roll.*

But Jeremy's bride wasn't prepared for such a commitment as marriage. Escaping the Midwest, she had sought sensation, not love. She embraced the thrill of a wedding and the spectacle of a Boston surprise. Too impatient for someone like Jeremy, for someone who believes deeply in loyalty and devotion, she wanted impetuous freedom; Jeremy yearned for fatherhood and a family home of his own.

It was less than a year until the bonds of marriage broke apart and they walked their separate ways, east of Eden. It was just a moment fading through time today, a distant memory, but not forgotten.

~

I have little understanding of what Dr. Shen meant when he said that he felt something in the soft muscles around the rectum when he examined Jeremy at St. Luke's—no understanding of that, no insight into what is lurking at the distant depths. And even more, I can't comprehend the enormity of what is developing right in front of us, right this minute, at Beth Israel.

Early Saturday morning, I'm still thinking Jeremy is going to be all right. Dr. Michael Groff, with his quick confidence and stark manner, enters the ER cubicle. Jeremy, exhausted, flat on his gurney, seeks relief.

About five feet nine inches tall, with a green sports jacket and matching tie, an alert smile on his youthful looking face, the neurosurgeon stands at the doorway, motionless for a moment. I have no idea who he is by status or reputation; I assume we still have time to talk about all this together, to decide what to do next.

Unaware that Groff's team is already gathering, preparing for surgery on the floor above us, Jeremy waits patiently to hear what Groff has to say; I am off balance as the doctor leans in.

"This is one of those moments," he begins. "A genuine emergency. Every minute makes a difference now."

It's as if he's started in the middle of the conversation. He's studied the MRI, but no one told me to expect this. What's he saying?

"We have to operate immediately. Get as much of the infection out of the spinal column as quickly as possible. Relieve the pressure on the cord."

Jeremy's face tightens; he's struggling with the doctor's words, as if the language itself is flowing, flooding over his sweating flesh. His eyes closed, he's absorbing what Groff is saying, but trying not to react.

Stop that talk. Slow it down, before we drown. Give it some time. "I'd like a second opinion," I blurt.

"I respect second opinions ordinarily, but no one would suggest anything else in this case, I assure you. And we don't really have the time."

Who is this guy? I wonder, gripping my cell phone in hand, clutching it tight, not knowing who to call to get information about this doctor, Michael Groff, about what is happening here. It's such an early hour, the sun just rising in the East at the beginning of the weekend.

Before I know it, Groff leans over Jeremy again, gazing down at him.

He starts to give Jeremy the grim facts: "There's about a thirty-three percent chance," he hesitates, "a thirty-three percent chance that you will come out of the operation the same as you went in."

Standing to the side, I can't believe what I'm hearing.

"Do you realize that he cannot walk now, that his legs are paralyzed?"

The surgeon nods, sensing my growing panic. He's resisting me, refusing to slow down: "And there is a thirty-three percent chance that you will be worse than when you went in."

Looking over at me, while Groff's words stir the air, Linda warns the room: "My husband is going to collapse."

My blood pressure drops, like a stone thrown into water. I spin, falling to the floor so I won't black out and drown. Suddenly it's as if I'm lying on hot sand, having been dragged from the shoreline. A kind young physician hands me a blanket to lie on and a metal container in case my body revolts, and I heave.

"Thank you," I respond, looking up at her, my throat parched, my voice barely audible.

And then I am somewhere else again, sensing the abjection, the liminal moment. Lying with eyes closed, I seem to be at a threshold, a dim border, unable to distinguish between the outside and the inside of my own baking skin. I listen to the rustling at the edge—the edge of a distant territory.

"We need a second opinion," I say when I begin to settle down. "What are you talking about? What do you mean 'worse'?"

"Well, I could stir something up around his spine. He could get meningitis," Dr. Groff answers in a measured tone. He focuses on Jeremy stretched across the gurney, but glances at me from the corner of his eye. Linda, clearly shaken, stands near the gurney, intent on the doctor's remarks.

The full ferocity of the turmoil is palpable for Jeremy now, the considerable weight of our voices pressing on him; he lies stunned. Next to his gurney Groff still looms down from above.

"You'll be okay, Jeremy," Linda promises. But Jeremy begins to sob, his body shaking, near hysterics. "Am I going to die?" he bellows. "Will I be paralyzed forever?"

The odds are not in his favor. We all realize that, as Groff suddenly departs, to ready for surgery upstairs.

When I gain my balance, I stumble out of the room, making my way to the nurses' station. I ask the same young physician who brought me the metal container a few minutes ago to find on her computer whatever she can about Dr. Groff. Who is this guy, I want to know, as I cast a forbidding shadow across her desk.

"And even if he does show signs of progress after the surgery, this does not mean he will recover fully," Groff indicated. "We just have to wait and see."

∼

The young doctor, the one who handed me the blanket, has found something of note about Groff. "Look at this," she says, pointing excitedly to the computer screen. Dr. Michael Groff, expert for neurosurgery of the spine at Beth Israel, the website indicates. Although young, Dr. Groff has built an impressive track record since becoming a physician in 1999. A rising star, he practices in one of the best hospitals in the country.

I run back down the corridor to tell Jeremy the news. "You're in good hands; Groff is an expert in this kind of operation. You'll be fine," I promise him. And, my feet now secure on the ground, I remind him how I have always delivered on my promise, remembering the time I lifted him up from his bed and carried him from room to room when he was a toddler frightened after a nightmare, promising him then that there were no monsters lurking in the house; and the time he couldn't sleep, the restless night before his driver's test, promising he would have his permit the next day, and sure enough, he did; and the time he wanted those Red Sox baseball tickets, promising I'd get some right behind the dugout, and the ancient usher sauntered down the aisle then and brushed off his seat with an old towel and welcomed him to the park. Yes, I am determined to deliver on this promise in the hospital as well, but all those previous promises seem so small and insignificant now.

Around 8:00 AM, an orderly enters the cubicle and wheels Jeremy out through the corridor to the elevator. They head upstairs to get ready for the medical team to prep him for the operation. Linda and I follow to the surgical vestibule where Jeremy lies surrounded by heavy, green curtains. Two anesthesiologists review their part in the procedure, asking Jeremy endless questions about his breathing, about his medical history, about his drug resistance. They gather needed information for their work in what we anticipate to be about a three-hour operation.

Then Dr. Groff appears again.

Linda immediately takes Groff aside. "There are no options here," she says. "We've already lost our oldest son, and we will not lose another. There is no option. Jeremy has to make a full recovery."

"You have to give Jeremy some hope," she continues, looking with penetrating eyes at Groff, her face reflecting her fierce mother love. "You can't bring him in there like that. This is intolerable. He's got to go into that operation with hope."

Staring straight at Groff, I respond to Linda's intensity; "I have great confidence in you," I tell him. "I know you're one of the top surgeons for the spine. You've got to be at your very best now." I look down at the floor for a moment, and then back up at him: "We refuse to accept any defeat here," I insist.

Dr. Groff acknowledges all this, nodding his head as I talk. Sensing I am done, he puts his hand on my shoulder, concerned about my unsettled behavior. "Not only will I do my best," he reassures me, "but better than anything I have ever done before."

Linda has left to be alone. Beyond Jeremy's sight, she leans sobbing against the corridor wall outside the vestibule area. An aide, who had been in the room with Jeremy, comes over to her, repeating over and over again: "I'm sorry. I'm so sorry." She too trembles with pain.

At that moment, Linda makes up her mind, calms her pounding heart. "I will be the head cheerleader on this journey, no matter how difficult it gets," she whispers to herself. "We must be optimistic. There is no other choice."

When Groff leaves the vestibule area for the operating room, I glance over at Jeremy as he looks up at me, his brave face forming a faint smile, a hint of terror at the edge. His body is rigid on the gurney; he seems to be holding his breath. As he is wheeled away, he turns his face once more toward me, and then he is gone, out of my line of sight, through doors, now closed, flat on the hard operating table.

∼

I pace up and down in the packed waiting area one floor above the operating room, my head bent low, my brown loafers scuffing the tiled floor. Other families gather in small groups, huddle in chairs or on couches and quietly chat to each other, trying to ease the passage of time. They too wait for news about their loved ones. One large group talks about their good friend who lost his leg in a motorcycle accident yesterday. Everyone appears bunched together, isolated in their own tight world.

So many hours I sat with Jonathan, our lost son, waiting. Waiting in the motel lobby in New York, waiting at Butler Hospital in Providence, waiting at Hazelden in Minnesota, waiting in the halfway houses, waiting at Roosevelt Hospital, waiting at LaGuardia Airport, waiting for his calls from California. I hoped never to hear the ringing of that final call, that call of death arriving without appointment at 4:00AM, that dreaded call ringing in the pitch dark, despite our optimism and hope, that call from the coroner with a southern accent on the West Coast.

"Is this Mr. Waxler."

"Yes."

"I am sorry but I have bad news."

"Yes."

"Your son Jonathan died tonight."

It was in the burst of a swirling snowstorm that Jonathan was born in 1969, the same year Neil Armstrong landed the *Eagle* near the Sea of Tranquility and then made the first moonwalk across that powdered charcoal landscape filled with ominous craters. "That's one small step for man, one giant leap for mankind," the astronaut said. Both Jonathan and Jeremy would come to know the meaning of that kind of dream walk. It helped define them, as they traveled together through time.

Born five and a half years later, in 1974, Jeremy is not as tall full grown as Jonathan at six feet, but his shoulders are broader than his older brother's, his back thicker. Always best friends, they inspired each other with their dreams. They sang songs and created exciting games together in the back seat of our car when we went on long family vacations. They shot hoops in our driveway, as if they were training to play for the Celtics; and they played catch on the grass in our backyard, preparing themselves for their inevitable appearance at Fenway Park. They were close. They were brothers.

Throughout those years, Jeremy was devoted to Jonathan, always listening with affection to his big brother's advice. He proudly smiled at Jonathan's passion and admired his struggle for social justice; he was impressed when Jonathan helped organize labor unions and when he committed his considerable energy to other worthy causes. Jeremy saw Jonathan as a kind and generous offshoot of the '60s: more Ken Kesey than Ozzy Osbourne; more Bob Dylan than Heavy Metal; more Easy Rider than Hells Angels. When Jonathan traveled quickly through college and then graduate school, Jeremy followed his every step.

And much later, when Jeremy witnessed firsthand Jonathan's torturous battle with heroin, he made it his battle, too. When Jonathan died, Jeremy was shattered by a pain that only a brother can understand, but he refused to give up hope. Later he would put it this way on his law school application:

> *Every day I think of the struggle of my brother, but I also reflect on the good fortunes of my own life. Although I have become increasingly pessimistic about the war on drugs and the future of many adults, I have become increasingly optimistic about the possibilities for finding meaning in the small acts of daily life. New chances and opportunities appear to me where I could*

never see them before. As a result, I try to make it easy for others to celebrate their lives. I try to be pleasant to everyone around me and treat everyone with respect because I am convinced that every human being deserves a chance to live a life of dignity and caring.

My own brother, David, who came with us from New Bedford to Beth Israel the night before, joins Linda and me while we wait in the family area for the call from Dr. Groff. The nurses have warned me, "It might take a while before the operation gets started, so don't worry if it's longer than three hours before the call comes." But I pace. I check the clock ticking on the wall. I fix on my watch, the brown leather band wrapped around my left wrist. I make idle conversation with Linda or David, but have little to say. I walk out of the main room into the outside corridor, return, sit down, get up, halt. What is happening to Jeremy, unconscious in the freezing operating room?

"It's taking much too long," I burst out, gazing over at Linda, then David, then back to Linda, specters floating in the air. "Groff should be done with the surgery by now," I claim.

I stare at the cell phone, looking at its small electronic screen. Have I missed the call? "He should have phoned by now," I insist again.

Dr. Groff finally calls around 1:20 PM. He says the surgery went well. The procedure lasted about two and a half hours, and now we just have to wait. Wait and see how the spinal compression subsides; how, as he puts it with a word that frightens me for weeks, the "crushed" spinal cord reacts to the insult it has endured. Wait and see how quickly the weakness in the legs and along the nerve circuits responds, how his toes move, if they do.

"Can you give me any sense of how this might develop?" I ask Groff, straining to hear some words of encouragement.

"No, I really can't. We just have to hope for the best."

Groff is always at a distance, cool and direct. Neurosurgeons protect themselves this way, I am sure. How else could they endure such pain and grief? On the front line day and night, perhaps they get used to the pain; perhaps they are just numb from the grief. How can any ordinary person stand such heartache, though? So real, so extraordinary. A bitter reminder of how fragile, how dangerous our lives really are.

Glancing out the hospital window, I am startled. In the far distance, I glimpse Jonathan, a boy miraculously falling from the sky.

> *"Father!" he cried as he fell, "Oh father, father, I'm falling!"*
> *Till the green of the wave closed on the agonized cry,*
> *While the father, alas, a father no longer, was calling,*
> *"Icarus, where do you fly, Icarus, where in the sky?*
> *Icarus!" he would call – and saw the wings on the water.*
> *Now earth covers his bones; now that sea has his name.* – Ovid

∽

Almost immediately after the operation, we are ushered into the Intensive Care Unit, the trauma center on the same floor as the operating room. Jeremy appears groggy but awake, unsettled but surprisingly healthy, the bed sheets loosely wrapped around him. Linda notes his energy right away. Although he can barely move, Jeremy gives us his broad smile—an effusion of joy, color in his face.

"He's a trooper," Linda says with genuine enthusiasm in her voice. She is optimistic, holding back her tears of gratitude and determined to cheer him on.

We are exhausted. We have not slept for two days, but Jeremy can wiggle his toes, and this is important. "You got through that, Jeremy," we all agree. "You're on the other side of it now."

"Yes, you're going to be fine," Linda adds, her tone at first focused like a laser beam, then soft and compassionate: "And Jonathan will be here to help you, too."

Yes, we have once again crossed that border where the ground trembles, and fear and hope swirl in the midst of the whirlwind. But where do we stand?

Protected by the twilight effects of the general anesthesia, Jeremy lies on his back in his bed, sensing little pain. He is well cared for by the attentive staff. They rapidly move in and out of his large hospital room, bringing medication, checking his vital signs and reading his charts and statistics. The room is one of several arranged in a semi-circle around the nurses' station. Monitors beep endlessly; screens dominate the space. Everyone is a marvel. But Jeremy can barely move.

Busy on her cell phone, one call after another, Linda rallies his friends and keeps them informed. I sit quietly in a wooden chair, making small talk with my son, while the afternoon shadows creep across the bed, forming strange patterns on the sheets. Jeremy dozes in and out of consciousness as the anesthesia begins to wear off. "I sure feel a lot better than yesterday," he says when he realizes how much time has passed.

As the natural light fades, we prepare to depart Beth Israel. We need to get some sleep. I kiss Jeremy on his forehead, Linda warmly hugs his body, and then we're in our car, headed home.

We glide along the highway, the radio playing soft music. Linda slumps over in the passenger seat, nodding off. Headlamps from the oncoming cars flicker by; the rhythm of the tires turning on the road soothes my body. When I tighten my grip on the steering wheel, my eyelids slowly close and then open with a start. I drift. Suddenly I am shouting aimlessly into the thick air, oblivious to the well-traveled highway in front of me. The light beams from our car splash on the night road, beckoning, pulling me further from myself. I am in a trance.

When we get home, Linda and I go directly to bed without much discussion. We are barely breathing.

∼

I awake from a sound sleep. Rising from our king-sized bed, I stagger out to the living room in the pitch black, warm tears falling along my cheeks. I bend my neck back to view the ceiling, soaring a lofty twenty feet above the floor, and then I yell again into the silence:

"They are trying to take him away from me, they are trying to take all that I have left in this world away from me."

The blast startles the quiet house, shakes the walls and frightens Linda asleep in the bedroom. Unhinged, I float free from all the gravity of ordinary life. I rave on the horizon of time.

Despite our sustained resistance since his brother Jonathan's death, we've returned with Jeremy to that place on the other side of health and security. It's very early Sunday morning, but from that incredible Friday evening on, I have sensed it, the shimmering and then the lightning bolt that changes perception and focus and finally brings the rustling of the cool wind. It is like a mirage rising from a valley of dry bones. All happening in the shudder of a moment.

We simply assumed a benign back pain when it started, a pain aching down through the legs, the result of pushing or pulling a large wooden dresser in his bedroom. We know better now. We assumed the obvious, and that assumption helped control our emotions, helped define the situation, helped falsify the truth. That assumption held us back from the edge for a while and kept us at a convenient distance. It could have cost Jeremy his life.

∽

They call it "an epidural abscess," an infection secretly crawling through the spinal column, eventually pressing, traumatizing, crushing the cord.

Spinal cord injuries occur in approximately 12,000 to 15,000 people per year in the United States. About 10,000 of these people are permanently paralyzed, and many of the rest die as a result of their injuries. Most cases of spinal cord trauma occur to young, healthy individuals. Males between fifteen and thirty-five years old are most commonly affected. Nearly 1.3 million Americans are living with a spinal cord injury.

For those attacked directly by an epidural abscess, the numbers are much lower, though the odds seem to remain about the same.

What can we do? Jeremy still has to endure a month-long regimen of intravenous antibiotics to be sure the infection is gone, but that's the least of our concerns. Will Jeremy ever be able to walk again? Will his bladder ever work again? Linda and I believe he will recover. We have to. But Dr. Groff appears less certain of that.

∾

At Beth Israel, Jeremy rests quietly. His face drawn, he remains groggy with little appetite. He's worried, but says little. If he's frightened, he keeps it to himself.

A young resident from Harvard sways into the room to check him and gently massage his weary flesh. Stunning and seductive, she stands before his bed, eager to do what she can to comfort him. Her big brown eyes catch his full attention. "It's difficult to know which nerves are working and which aren't," she says, her dark curly hair bobbing back and forth, her healing hands gently moving across his ailing back. "Those nerves all converge down here at the end of the spinal column," she explains, placing her fingers at the base of his spine and looking up toward his eyes. "They call it the horse's tail," the young doctor claims with a laugh when she is nearly finished.

After that, whenever he hears people pass by his door, Jeremy angles his face toward the corridor. He hopes to spot her and coax her back into the room.

"You might want to go out with her sometime," I mention to him, when I see his yearning.

He raises his eyebrows approvingly and chuckles, "Yes, that might be something to consider when I'm feeling better."

Later that afternoon, two staff nurses come into his room. "All right, Jeremy, we're going to get you out of that bed," they say, wrapping their arms around his trunk and holding him tight. With their help, he drags his body to the edge of the bed and sits up, placing both his feet on the floor. The nurses grab his underarms and pull his body forward, and as they do, he stands, gazing at us. Then, like a toddler, he takes four small steps, his face grimacing with raw desire and hope. I glance at Linda, whose eyes seem to open wide. Suddenly she jumps from her chair and throws her hands high in the air: "My son, oh my wonderful son," she shouts, filling the room with joy. She is amazed.

The following morning, Groff enters with his team, and they surround the bedside. The doctor shakes his head with approval, as he checks Jeremy, and, with his strange dry humor, the examination complete, he says to Jeremy:

"Okay, it's time. Get up and walk!"

It's a surprising remark, sending shivers along the spine, a sign of optimism, we believe—prophetic hope from the reluctant neurosurgeon. No doubt, Groff thinks it's going as well as it can. Dark clouds might linger around his brow, but he's impressed by what he sees.

"Okay, it's time. Get up and walk!"

His words ricochet around the walls and beckon to us from the shadows in the room.

"Arise, take up thy bed, and walk. And immediately the man was made whole, and took up his bed, and walked." That's what the Biblical text declares, describing Jesus's first miracle of healing.

Perhaps that's what Groff means; perhaps that's what we need now—a miracle. Is it possible?

Rehab

*H*is scarred body covered with a pale cotton hospital johnny, Jeremy prepares to depart Beth Israel by ambulance. He knows he's still alive, but he's uncertain, no longer sure about his place in the world. His body trembles, his back burns with pain. He has eaten little. He can barely stand. The paperwork complete, five days after surgery, he is ready to travel the sixty miles along the highway from Boston down the coast on Route 3 near Plymouth and then over the bridge to the RHCI—the Rehabilitation Hospital of the Cape and Islands in East Sandwich.

Right after the operation, I asked Dr. Groff where Christopher Reeve, the Superman of record, sought treatment after his catastrophe. I wanted to take Jeremy there when he was ready to leave Beth Israel. And then we considered bringing Jeremy to Spaulding in Boston, a well-known center for spinal cord treatment. But Groff didn't think any of this mattered.

"Just as well to take Jeremy to a place close to your home," he suggested. "All that special treatment Reeve received really didn't make a bit of difference. Those reports you've heard about, they really didn't mean anything. Reeve never recovered any significant movement—just twitches in his body."

The spinal cord will heal on its own, or not, the surgeon believes. And Linda's own doctor, a pain specialist from Cape Cod, agrees. She too has encouraged us to take Jeremy to RHCI.

So we are on our way, although we are not sure where we are headed.

We are on a long and treacherous journey, I imagine, deep in some other place. We are pilgrims and earth walkers, wandering in a strange land.

As I walked through the wilderness of this world, I lighted on a certain place where was a den, and I laid down in that place to sleep; and, as I slept, I dreamed a dream. I dreamed, and behold I saw a man clothed with rags, standing in a certain place, with his face from his own house, a book in his hand, and a great burden upon his back. I looked and saw him open the book and read therein; and as he read, he wept, and trembled; and not being able longer to contain, he brake out with a lamentable cry, saying, "What shall I do?" – John Bunyan

Pilgrims and wanderers. Earth walkers and dreamers. What shall we do?

∽

RHCI is a small, clean, well run rehabilitation center affiliated through Partners Corporation with the Boston medical network. Jeremy arrives first, and then, once we are there, a nurse brings the three of us to the second floor, where all the patients' rooms are located. The rooms line both sides of a long single corridor running the length of the building.

Jeremy shares his new room with a middle-aged man, average height, with short clipped hair and a slightly pudgy body. He suffered a tragic car accident a few days ago, when he was hit from behind by a drunk driver at high speed on the highway. His name is Pete. They tell us he has only a ten percent chance of ever walking again. Pete stares at the ceiling, barely able to move; his bones are splintered, his back broken. His fiancée sits in the wooden chair next to him. They stoically wait for the future to unfold.

"Jeremy, is it?" Pete asks when we get settled in the room. "Glad to meet you." When he hears Jeremy is making progress, his mouth curls into a smile; he's pleased at the news.

His life is devastated, his bones shattered; yet he lies there, refusing to yield. The skin below his eyes seems pale, sadly pulled down by the burden he bears, but the timbre of his voice lends dignity to the room and lifts the air around him. Although defeated, he is not destroyed, I see. He is wounded but not humiliated. Pete and his loving fiancée seem like a couple frozen in time, isolated in their own tenderness.

Several weeks later, long after Jeremy leaves the hospital, he will send Pete a card congratulating him on his wedding, although the ceremony will have to be conducted in the courtyard of the rehab center.

The staff at RHCI work three eight-hour shifts around the clock, and from Wednesday to Friday this first week, they hone in on Jeremy, checking him regularly. "Are you comfortable?" they want to know. "Do you want anything special to eat?" they offer. "We'll try some PT soon," they explain. Jeremy always nods his head with approval, anxious to get started.

The young doctor, Abramson, in charge of Jeremy's case (thirty-eight years old, dark hair, Jewish), the nurses and the aides, the physical therapists and the occupational therapists all appear compassionate and professional as they rotate through their positions each day, all rooting for Jeremy, fixing his bed covers, watching him closely and cheering him on.

∼

From the phone resting on a small table next to his bed, Jeremy calls each morning to give us an early report before we arrive to see him. Within a few days, he is settled into his new routine and sharply focused on his recovery; he believes he can spark that recovery with his will and determination. Using colorful magic markers, the staff posts a rigorous schedule for his exercises on a big board on the wall in the corridor. Friends send him get-well cards and text messages continually. His secretary at the law office checks in to see how he is doing, wishing quick recovery. Slowly, working very hard with the therapists for several hours each day, he gets his legs moving.

"I walked 100 feet today," he tells us in his enthusiasm on the phone. It turns out to be only twenty-five feet, leaning heavily on his metal walker and fighting his reluctant legs with each step, but his pride in the achievement is justified. The entire staff, delighted by this early and surprising success, warmly acknowledges us as soon as we arrive on the floor that day.

The nurse helps Jeremy into a wheelchair so he can sit up in his room for the first time. Satisfaction spreads across his face. His cheeks round with color, his back sturdy and erect against the hard metal, he is hungry with desire; he especially wants Linda and me to notice how well he is doing. Just watch me, he seems to be saying. I will not yield. I will return, make it all the way back.

> *I am the master of my fate;*
> *I am the captain of my soul.* – William Ernest Henley

But there's a battle going on, tremors of fear beneath his flesh. He might not make it back. Linda and I witness that battle, his strong will struggling against those rippling undercurrents.

He sits upright in the stiff wheelchair, but he sits there much too long, stubbornly resisting the nurse's command to return to his bed. "You're overdoing it," the nurse finally says as she responds to his rebellion.

When she bolts from the room, I take up her suggestion. "You're doing so well, Jeremy. Why not get back in bed now? You've been in that chair for at least two hours."

As the afternoon advances, his troubled body droops lower and lower in the chair; the bones of his spine begin to ache, as if they are turning to parched dust. Alone in his wheelchair, he refuses to listen to our voices; he looks only into our eyes. Linda and I serve as his mirror. As long as we acknowledge his achievement, progress will continue, he believes. He doesn't want to break that spell, and we don't want to disappoint him. But to me he is beginning to look haunted, like a ghost.

When he can't abide the pain any longer, he finally recants, thank goodness, reluctantly agreeing to get back in the bed. He realizes that he needs to limit such angry ambition.

While the nurse helps him back onto his mattress, he lets the breath out of his tense body.

Early the following day, another nurse, middle aged with straight, brown hair and children of her own, wheels Jeremy across the hallway to a vacant room. "You'll be next to the window," she explains with compassion. "Less noise from the busy corridor at night. A bed empty at least through the weekend."

"Yes, I like this room," he says, admiring the expansive space. "There's more sunlight, too."

He relaxes in his new room, reading the newspaper and sports magazines until his therapist takes him out to a large tiled space used exclusively for physical exercise. Supported by his aluminum walker, he shuffles 155 feet, making certain they measure each foot exactly so he can give us an accurate report. His legs still shake, his body unsteady, but his movement across the smooth floor is dramatic, offering promise these first few days, a rare delight—a miracle, some begin to believe.

∼

Jonathan was the first one in our family to see Jeremy walk. We were living in an apartment in New Bedford, and I was just starting out as a young literature professor. Raised in New Bedford, I felt rooted there; my parents were still living in the house I grew up in near Buttonwood Park in the West End of the city, and my brother was close by, only a few blocks away. We all had been part of that wonderful middle-class neighborhood. New Bedford, an ideal place to raise a family, I always thought. We had romped through those West End streets—Hawthorn, Plymouth, Carroll, Burns—and we had skated on the thick ice of the pond near the warming house in the park when we were growing up. New Bedford, the city where my brother and I had gone to public schools, the city that helped shape us, the Waxler family.

New Bedford, located in the southeastern corner of the state, right on the ocean. It had been an old whaling and textile town, and it still possesses a prosperous fishing port with rich ethnic neighborhoods and narrow streets with historic mansions. Some think of the city today as the gateway to Cape Cod. Others consider it an outmoded remnant of the old textile era, with its scarred "three deckers" crowding the neighborhood streets. For the Waxler family, though, it's always been our home turf. It whispers of the promise of the American Dream, of what the future can bring if only we can hear the rhythm of the city mingling with the roar of the ocean waves, calling passionately from the fine sand of the seashore.

Jonathan was six years old when he first saw his younger brother walk. "Come quick!" Jonathan yelled to Linda and me that morning: "I was holding Jeremy's hands in front of me, and I let him go. He took a step toward me all by himself before he fell. I know he'll get up again. Come quick."

Jonathan was so proud of his baby brother, the toddler then. Jeremy had gotten up on his own two legs. He had walked. If he had fallen, it didn't matter. He would get up again. That attitude flowed through the Waxler blood; it was rooted in the New Bedford soil.

Twenty years later, the summer after Jeremy's junior year at Tufts, he traveled with me to pick up Jonathan at Roosevelt Hospital in New York. It was Jonathan who had fallen this time. He had taken heroin, relapsed in the streets of the city, and was finishing up a ten-day stay for detox.

When we first saw him, Jonathan looked worn out but determined. "It's all going to be fine, now," he claimed in the hospital lobby. "I'll be back on my feet before you know it." It was the last time Jeremy would ever see his big brother.

New York was desolate that Sunday morning: the homeless, wrapped in tattered blankets, were sleeping against the brick walls of the hospital; litter was strewn on the streets from the festivities of the previous night. When the three of us ordered omelets for breakfast in a small restaurant across the street from the hospital, no one else was sitting at the tables. We should have driven home with him after breakfast, but we drove instead to LaGuardia Airport.

We waited a long time in those typical airport seats, the scratched and plastic ones, the kind that remind you how temporary and fragile the surface of the world has become. The airport buzzed and bustled with all sorts of people racing across the country that day. While we sat there, we talked about politics and literature, and Jonathan read some poems out loud—like this one from one of his favorite writers, Charles Bukowski, barfly and visionary:

> *don't be ashamed of*
> *anything; I guess God meant it all*
> *like*
> *locks on*
> *doors.*

Eventually his plane took off, floating for a few minutes in the blue sky, until that silver sphere disappeared, gone into the puffy clouds above us. Jonathan was in that plane, flying to a halfway house in California. Jeremy was by my side.

After that, Jeremy and I couldn't leave the airport terminal for a while. We stared at the posted schedules flickering on the electronic screens riveted to the walls, and we shuffled around but couldn't really move. It was as if our feet were stuck in cement. Finally, we broke free and walked straight out the airport doors, returning home to Linda. She was waiting for us in Dartmouth.

∼

Leaning over Jeremy's bed at the rehab center, Dr. Abramson, the dark-haired and handsome physician with a young family of his own, tells Jeremy: "We're going to start to retrain the bladder." When Jeremy left Beth Israel a week ago, his body was still essentially locked up, and his bladder remains so, inert, as if in a prison cell. "When will it work again?" Jeremy wants to know. He is beginning to walk, but his bladder is not functioning.

"Over the next forty-eight to seventy-two hours, the bladder should regain its flexibility and memory," Dr. Abramson claims. "This is not an uncommon situation."

Jeremy's right leg is not functioning normally either. In the big backroom where all the patients work out, Linda notices his leg drops when he walks as if it carries a heavy load, similar to the way it responded in his apartment just before his paralysis. Is this an early sign of a permanent limp? Dead weight that cannot be revived?

For me, the bladder becomes a central concern, and it disturbs Jeremy as well. Through hard work, Jeremy somehow might get control of his legs, a miracle in itself, no doubt, but he has no control of his bladder. It remains silent.

Linda refuses to discuss any of this. She believes that bright and colorful images, shaped and bounded by sunlight, will make everything all right. As she was when we last visited Jonathan in San Francisco, Linda insists on the optimistic cadence of reds and greens. But such rhythm occurs only at the surface of the skin, I imagine; tremors and turmoil swirl below. Vertiginous shadows dance at the border of the slanting light.

The troubled bladder looms. It evokes the possibility of a receding future: a catheter strapped to Jeremy's leg, a plastic bag dragged with his body; a permanent attachment to his life weighing him down, narrowing his movement. It nags and nags at me.

I wonder which is worse, the wheelchair or the catheter in this distorted context.

∽

Jeremy's unsteady legs, his aching spine, his inert bladder, his very identity, all are organically connected to each other, the literature professor thinks. The human body extends out into the world and moves through it; language gives that body meaning and direction.

I am reading up on the American Transcendentalists for my undergraduate seminar in the fall semester. Thoreau, the sage from Walden Pond, knew something important about Jeremy's condition:

Methinks that the moment my legs begin to move my thoughts begin to flow—as if I had given vent to the stream at the lower end and consequently new fountains flowed into it at the upper.

Exactly. The legs move, the body flows, and the words spill from our lips as we meet the world, coming and going.

"Walking is a crusade." That's what Thoreau says in his essay "Walking," and I'll be sure to let my students know. We're all on a journey, I'll tell them. Free men and women, sauntering and open to the wildness. Not the wilderness but *the wildness*. My students will like this essay, I think.

We can all be earth walkers, seeking the natural flourishing of the whole body. As we journey forward, we meet the wildness of the world and as we go, we interpret the language of nature unfolding before us. That is what I will say to my students.

That wildness, that flow, is what Jeremy seeks, too. I see his yearning reflected in his light bright eyes when he looks up from his bed at me.

Yes, Thoreau's essay reads me as much as I read it. We are always reading ourselves when we read each other.

Am I dreaming?

I have always believed that literature and life intersect, that language and stories give our experience meaning. Back in 1991, I shared this belief in the power of literature with a friend, Judge Bob Kane, who, at the time, was concerned with "turnstile justice," as he put it. "Literature can make a difference, Bob," I told him after a tennis match that August summer. "Take eight men coming before your bench headed back to jail," I suggested, "and sentence them instead to a literature program at the university. I'll get the seminar room, choose the books, lead the discussion. I bet it'll change their lives."

That was the beginning of one of the projects that gives me the most pride, an experiment which continues now in eight states and in England and which has had remarkable success in reducing recidivism rates and shaping the lives of thousands of readers from all walks of life. Called "Changing Lives Through Literature" (CLTL), the program demonstrates how literature and life are interwoven.

We create our own stories, our own life, if we are fortunate. Stories we read help us to locate ourselves in the world, help us to find ourselves amidst the other stories and voices we hear and see. As the contemporary philosopher Richard Kearney once put it: "The unnarrated life is not worth living."

One night, a CLTL student insisted on telling all of us around the table about his experience with Santiago, the old man in Ernest Hemingway's story.

There he was, the student explained, walking down Union Street (a main street in New Bedford), ready to make a turn back to his old neighborhood after struggling to remain clean from drugs for some time. Suddenly he heard the voice of Santiago calling to him, reminding him of what the old man, with his wounds and scars, had suffered through, what the vulnerable old fisherman had heroically endured. Santiago was an inspiration to him, encouraging him to walk straight down Union Street, not to turn away. "Santiago saved me, at least for that day," the student wanted us to know. He was no longer alone; a character from literature had become a friend, a bosom buddy.

At their best, I believe, all stories have this kind of ethical standing. They can redeem us, soothe us at times, perhaps even keep us from the sting of death itself. A shared story serves as a covenant that binds us together and calls to us.

A shared story is a promise offering hope.

The poet Auden put the matter this way:

About suffering they were never wrong,
The Old Masters; how well, they understood
Its human position; how it takes place
While someone else is eating or opening a window or
just walking dully along;

It's just about a week since Jeremy began his ordeal. His five-foot-ten-inch frame is prone on the hospital bed. He, too, is dreaming.

He imagines a sun-drenched June morning outside Dartmouth High School a decade ago, the grass finely cut, families sitting in the stands in colorful shorts and shirts. As he mounts the stairs to the podium, eager to receive his high school diploma, he holds tight on his head a green graduation cap with a gold tassle. The cap barely fits on his big, round skull; his left hand struggles against the wind to keep that cap in place. With Linda at my side, I look down at the graduation program, proud to see Jeremy's name in the top five percent of the class. When I look up, the principal, near the microphone, holds Jeremy's diploma and announces his name, "Jeremy Regan Waxler." That name bellows through the loud speakers, circling through the stadium, swirling through the hearts of all those who care about him—so many proud and determined parents gathered together, hearing that name, Jeremy Regan Waxler, on that joyful day.

In his bed, Jeremy's eyes remain shut. He dreams about all his wonderful friends on the small liberal arts campus at Tufts. He saunters with those young students over the green grassy hills in springtime, hills covered with a napkin of white snow in winter. He calls to Esteban, now a lawyer in D.C.; to Nicole, now a publisher in Boston; to Dara, now a financial analyst on Wall Street; to Mark, now a physician at Hasbro Children's Hospital in Providence; to Luke, now a business executive; and Dennis, his good buddy from Cape Cod, now an insurance adjuster. They all shout back to him, their voices echoing through the campus green: "Hurry up, Jeremy. Get better soon."

Motionless on his bed, Jeremy imagines and imagines. He is in flight now to the brick courthouse where he served as an assistant district attorney in Bristol County, south of Boston. He hears the hectic rhythm of the courtroom: the clerk's shout, the judge's gavel, the jury filing into the box. He is determined and energetic as he makes his legal arguments before the bench. He balances the scales of justice with mercy and with memories of his beloved older brother, whom he refuses to ever forget. The court officers address him as "counselor" as he walks through the corridors; he nods back at them with pleasure as he passes.

I once saw Jeremy at a pre-trial hearing in Fall River District Court when he was still a prosecutor for the government.

The notorious rapper Busta Rhymes had been accused of assault in a Fall River bar after a concert, and the courtroom was packed with fans and the media. Rhymes chatted with his New York lawyer by his side, the big city attorney dressed in a blue pin-striped suit and bright tie. Rhymes' Boston lawyer, a man well known for his charm, was also there that morning, glad-handing the court officers. Behind closed doors, Jeremy negotiated with these lawyers and with Rhymes himself for about an hour while the restless crowd buzzed with anticipation. Then the lawyers emerged from the room and stood before the judge's bench in open court. Jeremy had settled the matter, and the ruling was announced: six months probation and a fine for Rhymes. Everyone seemed satisfied. A balance had been struck. Rhymes went out to meet the media. "I guess I'm just too sexy...buy my albums," the rapper said, playing to his excited fans outside the courthouse. Jeremy, the attorney of record, slipped out the back door, back to his office to work on his next case.

Yes, Jeremy is a man of principle and a talented lawyer. He doesn't seek the limelight, but you can always call on him to come through. When my younger brother, David—an established New Bedford attorney with a prosperous practice in personal injury law—needed to replace an associate who had recently quit the firm, he called on

Jeremy. Three years ago. "I think it's time for you to leave the DA's office. Come work with us. It'll be a good change of pace, and you'll make more money," my brother suggested. David knew Jeremy was a good lawyer, that Jeremy was always eager to take a case to trial, was amiable and a quick learner. David needed Jeremy, and Jeremy needed the experience in civil practice and in a private office. The change was good for both of them.

Stretched out on his hospital bed now, Jeremy remains quietly determined. He'd like to get back to his friends and to work.

∼

Five of Jeremy's good buddies, young and restless, surround him by his bedside at the rehab center, chatting about the Red Sox, local politics, the beaches and the parties. What they are saying doesn't matter as long as they say it, language creating a dwelling for friendship. These young men are good friends of my son, and they have come to visit him in his time of need. Jeremy is caught, whirling in the warm flow of their laughter and talk as they crowd close to his bed. They make his round cheeks radiate with joy, raising his hope high with their exuberance and energy.

A few hours later they are gone, and Jeremy, alone with Linda, his mother, reflects on the day, as shadows begin to slip across his room. His body is covered with a white sheet, only his brave face exposed to the cool air. When I enter the room from the corridor, I gaze over at Linda, my beautiful and optimistic wife, standing close to his bed, and then I see Jeremy, his cheeks stained with tears. He turns his head toward me, startled, as if he has seen a ghost. Immediately he draws the sheet up above his face. He is hiding, out of my sight. He does not want his father seeing him this way. He needs to keep this part of his struggle secret from me, draw a border between us, a clear line I should not cross.

Later that evening, he regains his composure and balance. "I can't believe what a baby I was before," he says, shaking his head in disgust.

"You're no baby," I tell him. "You're just human like all of us. I can't believe how well you are doing."

~

Each morning before dawn, I awake and wander alone through the darkness hanging heavy like a shroud in the silent house. I stop and take a drink of cool water in our kitchen and listen, hearing the refrigerator humming, the painted clock ticking on the shelf. Then, with my bare feet on the wooden floor, I roam across the living room and lay my head on the pillow, soft and puffy, resting there on the easy chair next to the fireplace until I grow tired. Curled tight in that cushioned seat, I finally rise and return to Linda in our king-sized bed, completing the circle of my night journey.

Lying next to Linda, her eyes quiet with sleep, I stare up at the ceiling and picture Jeremy in his bed; he is waiting, as I am, for the future to unfold. He is restless and uneasy, imagining what has not yet arrived.

I doze off, just when the early morning light breaks, streaming into the room through the closed curtains.

Where are You, God? I'd like to know. Do you remember Your Promise? Do you remember Your Covenant?

I shall bless you abundantly and make your descendants as numerous as the stars in the sky or the grains of sand on the seashore. – Genesis 22:17

Are You present in that morning light blazing through the drawn curtains covering Jeremy's window? You know his fears: that he will never be whole again, never be able to party with his friends on a Saturday night, never walk through the courtrooms that he loves, never bear children. I would change places with him in a second if You would offer me that opportunity. But what parent wouldn't?

There are people worse off than Jeremy: Pete, his old roommate, for example, lying on his broken back in his hospital bed, barely able to move; Jonathan, resting silently in his grave.

But right now, I think only about Jeremy. Some say I am obsessed.

And what do people expect? I can only try to sew the thin thread of hope back through his body. Faith without evidence—that is what faith is. It is a promise, a dream.

Time unfolding with all its terror will somehow work in our favor. We have to believe this.

∼

Late Saturday night, I sit in a chair on the large wooden porch in the back of my home, overlooking the tree-lined valley below. It's a warm night; flies buzz in the darkness. Numerous stars twinkle against the sky, abundant like grains of sand on the seashore. With my eyes shut in the darkness, I fly from my lounge chair to the brightest star. In the quiet breeze, as I go, listening to the hum of the busy beetles, I hear all the well intentioned phrases that people are mouthing in the wind: "Keep positive and optimistic," they assert; "Hold onto the good faith," they say; "Believe and he will be just fine," they insist; "It could have been worse," they think. But their words are like empty chatter to me. I cannot listen to them for long. They are drawing a borderline as a defense. Their voices float at the surface as they pass by.

On the stained-wood porch, I dwell, listening in the darkness, and I am delivered to the place Linda discovered after Jonathan died. Her advice then is all that I can hear now: "Let just a little in at a time," she said in the midst of our common grief. Let just a little in at a time, like a sliver of moonlight slipping through the clouds.

Perhaps Linda's advice offers the best approach now.

I don't think so, though. I refuse that call.

∼

A smudged, plastic nametag fastened around his wrist, Jeremy lies on his back in his $18,000 hospital bed, a technological marvel at the Cape Cod rehab center. What merit and meaning does all that high-powered investment have? It is only a pretense of modern control. Jeremy simply wants to turn his quivering body in that bed and gain some slight comfort. He struggles on his own. His bare hands fumble until he gets a tight grip on the cold metal side bar of that modern marvel. He works alone, his fingers clutching that bar. His palms press against the metal while he calls up all the strength he can muster from his battered limbs. He wants to lift his heavy trunk from the mattress; he wants to log-roll over and rest on his side. It is a challenging job, and all the sophisticated technology in the world cannot help him.

It was so easy for him just a week or so ago. He didn't think twice then. Bounding out of bed in his apartment, he leaped onto the firm floor, his bare feet blowing like a gust of wind across the room. Roaring to the kitchen, he grabbed onto a pan from the shelf, cracked three eggs and fired up a mouth-watering omelet.

On Sunday morning, only nine days since the surgery, Jeremy is elated when he calls: "I walked 300 feet this morning, leaning on the metal walker."

Linda and I embrace.

Still very wobbly, he stands upright without assistance. "I did it this morning," he says. "I stood on my own two legs in front of the mirror above the sink. And then I saw my face reflected in that glass. I was steady; I had balance. I lifted my left arm slowly, and then—it was difficult, but I brushed my teeth."

∼

When Linda and I arrive at his rehab bed early Sunday afternoon, Jeremy greets us with a rejuvenated tone of success in his voice: "I feel lighter," he says, "less bloated." And he looks relieved, his body delivered, his eyes dancing.

By suppertime, he is gobbling down a jumbo lobster roll and crispy french fries with ketchup, which I bought for him at Captain Scott's, an old traditional seafood restaurant down the road from the hospital, off of Route 6A. A rambling oceanside place with formica tables and friendly waitresses, Captain Scott's is an authentic destination, patronized and enjoyed by Cape Cod families for many generations.

"I didn't want to eat much before," Jeremy explains, sitting with his empty tray in front of him. "Just worried about stuffing my insides." Now he seems ready, eager to root himself into the rhythm of the old traditional pleasures, ready to return soon to the Venus de Milo restaurant in Swansea for another lobster celebration, a birthday feast, I begin to believe.

At home that night, I search the Internet for information about John of God; I'm considering a trip to Brazil if Jeremy can't get the bladder started, or if he needs an additional charge to stimulate his back and legs. Thought by many to be the most powerful medium and healer in the world today, John is a phenomenon, and I've been intrigued by him for several years. Supposedly, at his remote countryside compound in Central Brazil, John channels through his body the greatest surgeons that every lived. In that compound, he has thirty surgeons on call, some living and some dead; they touch thousands of patients each day. Among those luminaries are Dom Inacio de Loyola, a fifteenth-century Spanish nobleman; Dr. Oswaldo Cruz, who helped to eradicate yellow fever; and the late Dr. Augusto de Almeida, a meticulous and demanding surgeon.

Dr. Mehmet Oz, Professor of Cardiac Surgery at Columbia University, defends John: "Crawfish regrow their nerves, right? Maybe there are things that we could harvest in our psyche that allow us to do it as well."

I'd travel to see John in a minute if I thought he could heal Jeremy. I'd like to witness his work before Jeremy leaves the rehab center, and then, if needed, take Jeremy to Brazil.

Others continue to believe I am crazy, of course. They think that I've already flown to another country; they claim that I'm exploring the terrain of weird tales. But there are always strange stories, as strange as the surreal night at Beth Israel when Jeremy, paralyzed, lay helpless on his gurney, and I fell to the ground, unable to walk.

At the Dartmouth Woods apartment complex, where Jeremy ordinarily lives, I hear the tale of a young man, about thirty years old, struck down in Fall River. Rushed to the hospital, he died within a half hour from what was diagnosed at first as EEE (triple E, as they call it), but now they claim it was spinal meningitis. All this supposedly happened a week or so ago. I should investigate further, get the names and details of this strange case—pass that information along to the infectious disease team at Beth Israel, although that team can't discover any cause for Jeremy's own strange infection.

It seems coincidental, weird, but it needs pursuit. Unravel this mystery that came on like a surprising summer storm. I don't want it ever to occur again. We need to expose it, give it a name, and make sure it never returns.

Is that crazy?

~

Jeremy blooms in the morning sun. His metabolism seems smooth and balanced at those hours, energetic, his serotonin levels high. He is bright and beaming then. At dusk, the disease demons appear, dancing like shadows on the hospital wall. He is melancholy, at times lonely, irritable. Twilight hints at the darkness, seeks out the hollow spaces in the spinal column. His motion stifled, his freedom inhibited, Jeremy asks: "Will I ever be able to have children?" He'd like to know.

He was fortunate to have the hospital semi-private room to himself through the weekend, but now they have put another patient in the bed next to him, a middle-aged man with low tolerance for noise, suffering from a fall from a bicycle that caused temporary brain damage. The man should have worn protective headgear on the road, I suppose. It might have made a difference.

His wife and son come to visit him during the day. While sleeping, Jeremy's new roommate snores throughout the dark night.

We move Jeremy to a private room at the far end of the hospital corridor. Quiet and comfortable, he begins a new regimen of drugs to stimulate the nerves and muscles in his unresponsive bladder. His staff physician, Abramson, reads as hopeful all the signs from the bladder.

"Why are you so optimistic?" I ask Dr. Abramson.

"Partly because the nerves running into the bladder are lower on the spinal cord than the nerves most directly affected by the infection. And partly because of Jeremy's remarkable progress so far."

As another doctor will tell me much later, sounding as if he were Thoreau: "As the feet go, so goes the bladder."

∼

Lightning never strikes the same place twice, they claim. But I disagree. Jonathan died on August 20, 1995, at the age of twenty-six; we are approaching twelve years since his death. We traveled then in the midst of a bitter wind, never expecting anything like that to happen again in our family. Lightning never strikes twice, they say. But they are wrong.

I remember how Linda was in her grief, her silent mourning for Jonathan. So quiet. She refused to return to teaching high school. She was somewhere else. Her nerves ached. Her gall bladder almost exploded. She developed fibromyalgia. She rarely picked up the phone to speak.

Linda needed that isolation to survive. Now I rarely talk to anyone. I hesitate to answer most phone calls, or make them, unless they offer signs of progress on the path we are traveling with Jeremy.

But I don't want to discourage Jeremy, and Jeremy is in the worst place of all.

Perhaps all we can do is wait. There's virtue in that, the poet Milton wrote: "And they also serve, who only stand and wait."

But the poet was reflecting on his blindness when he composed that line.

Bounding through the front door of RHCI early Wednesday afternoon, Linda and I immediately spot Jeremy's physical therapist, the one he especially likes. Always upbeat, multi-colored with tye-dye flashes of brilliance, she reminds him of Jonathan, a hippie from some other world.

Her hazel eyes shimmer as she stands by the staircase in the lobby, her hands on her hips, her slim body slightly tilted, her weight resting on her right leg. Keen joy rises in her voice: "Jeremy is doing so well. He walked with a cane today. Walked up several stairs, too. He's pushing his body out to the limit," she insists. "And when we talked about how lucky he was to be going to your house, he laughed about your cooking skills."

But then we climb the stairs to the second floor, where all the patients stay, and the world twists again. Jeremy looks distraught. He's running a temperature above 100 degrees, and the fever climbs higher throughout the day. A dangerous infection, I think, the return of a monstrous bacteria ransacking his injured spine.

Nurses prepare a series of blood cultures to check for bacterial infection. They puncture his skin with syringes, draw blood from inside his body and place the vials in their neat plastic kits. Then they need a picture of his abdomen. They wheel him downstairs to the x-ray room, a barren place except for the machinery—looming like a lonely robot hanging from the ceiling—and the long metal table in the middle of the floor. The nurses gently guide him onto the table. He lies against the hard surface, his troubled back burning with fire, until they get the pictures they require. When they are done, he is returned to the second floor, back to the comfort of his bed.

In the afternoon, Linda and Jeremy read some of the many get-well cards he has received, while I drift out to the hospital lounge. "He is too young for this to happen," I whisper, slumping down in an easy chair, my eyes darting back and forth across the empty room. Suddenly I hear Jonathan rustling in the distant corner.

I'm glad I came out to the lounge. I don't want Jeremy seeing me at such an edge. He scrutinizes the wrinkles in my face, whether they twinkle or twitch; he seeks signs of his condition in each quiver of my body. When I mirror sadness, he flinches.

Jeremy's blood tests prove negative, but I don't calm down for a while. "Well, you were better later in the day, Dad. I guess you can come back tomorrow," Jeremy half-jokingly says at the end of the day.

But he is cranky, and his nurse seems slow moving and slow thinking as dusk settles in. "The nurse from hell," we later dub her.

Later that night, Jeremy calls the house: "I am feeling better," he tells Linda. "And a different nurse came in to catheterize me. She did a great job. No pain," he says. "I hope she'll take care of me from now on."

Just imagining his upbeat voice rejuvenates me. My emotions so tightly tied to his right now, his relief is mine as well.

I bring a novel—*Saturday* by Ian McEwan—to read the following day, so I won't hover over him. The novel turns out to be about unexpected trauma in the family and about Henry Perowne, a neurosurgeon whose life is suddenly turned upside down on a weekend:

> *Henry can't resist the urgency of his cases, or deny the egotistical joy in his own skills, or the pleasure he still takes in the relief of the relatives when he comes down from the operating room like a god, an angel with glad tidings—life, not death.*

Thinking he is neatly wrapped in privilege, Dr. Henry Perowne believes he is safe and secure, but, as he discovers, he clearly isn't. Who is? There is no safe place.

∼

I need to do something, anything to feel I'm helping Jeremy progress.

I call my urologist at Massachusetts General Hospital and get the name of the leading neurourologist there, Pablo Gomery. He has nothing available for Jeremy until September, and although I wish the good doctor could do something right away, I hope the bladder will regain its natural rhythm and coordinate its nerves and muscles even before Jeremy leaves the rehab center. Then, there will be no need for

Dr. Gomery at all. We reserve the appointment for late September, almost two months away, already into autumn, just in case.

Then I barrage the affable Dr. Abramson, although I see he's growing tired of hearing my voice. "How long can Jeremy take those new pills for his bladder?" I ask him. "Can we use that medicine at home?" I want to know. "How long does it usually take for them to take effect?" I wonder. "Should we try to stimulate the bladder with acupuncture? The Chinese use that method," I continue.

The doctor is patient and understanding: "I make rounds early each morning at dawn," he jokes. "Perhaps you should join me then? You can ask your questions as we go."

Yes, he maintains good humor, as they all do, and I persist. I know how annoying this can be, how impulsive it is, but what can anyone expect from parents who have lost one son and refuse to lose another? And where do you draw a reasonable line that separates obsession from compassion anyway? "What is now reason was formerly impulse," the Greek poet Ovid said. I'll be sure to tell my students that next semester.

∼

On Thursday, fewer than two weeks after his surgery, the doctors begin to prepare for Jeremy to leave rehab. He'll be in our house the beginning of next week.

"It'll be like I am back in high school," Jeremy claims. He doesn't want to return to those nostalgic glory days of adolescence. At our house, he'll feel as if he is back-peddling, while time irrevocably moves forward. At thirty-three years old, he needs an opening, "a clearing," as the philosopher Heidegger would put it.

When Dr. Groff offered up those frightening odds in the emergency ward at Beth Israel, Jeremy was struck with terror. But later, when Groff suggested he might have to go home with his parents for a while, Jeremy burst out in revolt. "That's not going to happen," he insisted. "I'll be just fine in my apartment. I can take care of myself." Our son doesn't want to return to his parents' house, but he has no choice. He needs his body healthy for gravity and direction; he needs a dwelling place for protection and guidance.

Granted, Jeremy has traveled a long distance from that first night at Beth Israel, when his feet felt like stone in the hour of lead. Emily Dickinson described it this way:

> *The Feet, mechanical, go round—*
> *Of Ground, or Air, or Ought—*
> *A wooden way*
> *Regardless grown,*
> *A Quartz contentment, like a stone.*
> *This is the Hour of Lead—*
> *Remembered, if outlived,*
> *As Freezing persons, recollect the snow—*
> *First—Chill—then Stupor—then the letting go.*

Jeremy has progressed through that hour of lead, but he still struggles for location. He has a significant way to go. We all do.

Not quite two weeks since his operation, time seems to move so slowly—and I seem empty of everything but Jeremy's illness.

And what if he were married with a wife and children? What if he had his own comfortable home to return to—his own dwelling place, safe and secure? Those are his dreams. They would make for a different story, a different journey and a different life, I see.

The case worker—a slim and energetic woman about forty years old with short-cropped hair and dimples in her cheeks—begins the difficult job of organizing Jeremy's transition. Professional and efficient, she lines up the physical therapist, the occupational therapist, and the home health care nurses. She talks with the insurance provider; she orders the intravenous paraphernalia and a full box of catheters.

When we enter her office, papers scattered all over the desk, she swivels around in her chair: "Officially, Jeremy will be allowed only three days for the nurses to run the intravenous set up at your place," she says. "That's all the time the insurance will grant you. After that, you'll have to learn to adjust the lines and the machinery on your own."

"How do they make such judgments?" I ask, shaking my head in response and thinking about all the trouble we faced fighting the insurance company when Jonathan was in jeopardy. "We actually don't believe in rehab for you druggies," some bureaucrat told Jonathan once on the phone.

Jonathan was calling from his detox bed then, trying to arrange his next move toward recovery. "Rehab doesn't work—especially for heroin addicts," they told him. Jonathan was a man seeking help, fighting for his life, but they only offered him cost ratios.

"The insurance bureaucrats from hell," we dubbed them later.

∼

On Friday, Jeremy returns to physical therapy, as if everything were normal. At the edge of the large exercise room, I watch from a distance as the patients, young and old, struggle to regain their stamina. Some work with pulleys to strengthen their arms or legs. Some stretch out on a blue plastic mat. Others roll, back and forth, on a big, bright red ball. Jeremy leans on his walker as he moves across the room, his muscles flexing, almost fluent now. He seems faster than the therapist who pretends to have trouble keeping up with him when he scuffs across the smooth tiled floor. His eyes are raised to the distance before him. He laughs, picking up speed for a while. Then his feet begin to drag. Enough for today.

Later Linda and I take Jeremy in his wheelchair through the busy rehab corridor to play scrabble on one of the big, round tables in the recreation area. He calls to Pete, who twists his head toward him as we go, and then, down the corridor, we settle in the game room. Other patients sit quietly there with their families and friends, gathered in tight units, playing cards and checkers, some munching on fresh chocolate chip cookies. When we unfold the scrabble board on the table and smooth it down, Jeremy's flesh brightens, his breath flows from his skin like a gentle breeze filling the summer air. The three of us take turns around the table, each making words from the letters on our plastic tiles. We place those tiles on the colorful squares of the game board and then record our scores on a small pad of paper.

By dinner time, Jeremy has worked up an appetite, and with Linda sitting by his side, he eats Salisbury steak and mashed potatoes with brown gravy and peas. Outdoors, in my shirtsleeves, I stand on the asphalt in the parking lot, talking on my cell phone to Adrian Gardner, Jeremy's infectious disease physician at Beth Israel.

"We're closing out our investigation," Dr. Gardner tells me. He's preparing to leave his office for the weekend. "About thirty to forty percent of the bacterial infection cases like Jeremy's remain mysterious, never resolved," the doctor explains.

Gardner believes some kind of common bacteria got into the spinal column through the blood stream and then sought an empty space to settle. Once the bacteria mushroomed, that mass pressed against the cord and damaged the nerves.

"It's uncommon but we see it happen," Gardner claims. "These bugs are strange. They seek hollow places in the body. That's why you might get a strep throat, for example. The spinal column is an unusual destination for bacteria, but it's a hollow space."

"What about his bladder?" I finally ask Gardner. But the doctor says what they all say: "No way to tell about this right now. You just have to wait it out and hope."

Back upstairs, empty dinner plates rest on the bed tray; Linda and Jeremy listen to the television hanging on the far wall. They look beaten down. But when Jeremy's nurse arrives in the room, she's smiling: "I've got exciting news," she says. "Starting tonight you can get up yourself whenever you want to." Jeremy nods with approval, but he doesn't say anything. Still determined, he's ready to fight, but he's not willing to get too excited. He's keeping a distance from his emotions.

We take his walker from the corner of the room and place it near his bed, in case he decides to try to walk on his own. Jeremy watches in silence. He seems uneasy but resolute. He'll try the walker, I am sure, when he is alone and no one can see him.

Around midnight, I picture Jeremy leaning against that walker in the middle of his rehab room. His eyes shut, he considers the long journey from his bed to the bathroom. Is it worth it right now? Alone in the darkness, he trembles, dreaming about his young pals spilling surplus energy as they roar with laughter throughout Cape Cod. He sees his friends traveling together, hoisting their beer mugs at club after club. Are they thinking about me? Jeremy wonders, as his metal walker scrapes across the hospital floor.

Not a party animal, Jeremy often likes to stay home and relax, watch television or a movie from Netflix. But he misses the freedom to choose his own path, yearns now for the gift of free movement, for the ability to travel from place to place without hindrance.

And then I see Jeremy again, phoning us from his apartment about two weeks before his paralysis: "My lip is all swollen. All of a sudden, for no reason."

"You should take some Benadryl," Linda tells him. She imagines the swelling is an innocuous allergic reaction. "Let's wait and see what develops."

A few hours later the swelling subsides, mysteriously disappearing, just as it mysteriously arrived. Back to normal.

A hint at the origins of his infection? A clue to the start of that strange and disturbing rumbling of the body? The first sign of that ghostly bacteria fleeing into his blood stream, pushing across the border, haunting the hollow space inside his spinal column? The weird bug, unnamed and mysterious, revealing itself?

Perhaps the horror first entered his body when he vacationed in Brazil with his friends a few months ago.

∽

Near the end of the weekend, Jeremy eagerly anticipates a visit from another group of friends, four good buddies from the New Bedford area. These friends have called from a cell phone in their SUV. Like young rebels, they're traveling together along the road, driving near the Cape Cod Canal to the rehab center. They are movers and shakers in the community, young lawyers, assistant district attorneys with good political radar. They will be county commissioners, state legislators, perhaps even trial court judges one day.

"I've got to get the nurse," Jeremy says when he puts down the phone. "I'll need her to work the catheter before they arrive." He's anxious, not wanting his friends to think about his bladder. "They'll have to wait outside my room," he insists, realizing the nurse at his bedside will have to drain his bladder and measure the results with her electronic scanner before they see him.

About half an hour later, his buddies pull into the hospital parking lot. They are dressed in lightweight slacks and button-down shirts, and they emerge from their car like a friendly and energetic gang of politicos. They bound up the long flight of stairs, two steps at a time, to the second floor to see our son. They are good friends to Jeremy. Their camaraderie and high spirits flare as they joke with each other, joyfully pushing and shoving along the rehab corridor.

Knowing they are eager, his nurse discreetly works the catheter behind closed doors. His friends gather on the other side of that door, in the hallway, bantering about work and community affairs—and, of course, about Jeremy.

Linda and I join them as they wait, and I stir their attention with details of Jeremy's experience that first night at Beth Israel. Surprised and riveted by what I'm saying, they listen intently, the words flowing from my lips.

I give them the odds Groff gave us.

"Thirty-three percent chance he would be no better and no worse; thirty-three percent chance he would be worse; thirty-three percent chance he would improve, but that didn't necessarily indicate he would ever walk again. Those are the brutal statistics the surgeon gave Jeremy that night when he hovered over him like a helicopter," I explain. "It was traumatic, Jeremy lying on that gurney."

His friends shuffle about near the couches in the hallway. Shaken, they look at each other, then at me: "We didn't realize all this. It's much worse than we imagined."

Inside the enclosed room, the nurse works quickly while Jeremy lies flat on his bed. Torn between his need for his overbearing parents on the one side and his desire for meaningful work and trusted friends on the other, he acknowledges now he will live at our house for at least a month when he leaves the rehab center.

In his head, he maps out what he will need, what he will do, how he will manage and negotiate through the long, drawn-out days with us. He'd like to get out of his drab hospital gown, strip naked, wrap his body in bright-colored garments and return to his own spacious apartment. But he knows right now he has no choice. He'll stay with us until he completes his intravenous treatment, and then, if he's fortunate, he'll be set free.

At our house, he will require a strict schedule for his intravenous drip (twice a day); for the heavy dose of antibiotics to protect his body from infection; for the physical therapist (three times a week); for the occupational therapist, if necessary; for his heparin shot each morning to prevent blood clots; and for the self-catheterization to empty his bladder (four to six times a day).

But, for the moment, Jeremy is finished with the nurse, and the door to his room is thrown open. His friends rush in, greeting him with all the thrill and excitement of young vitality and restless desire.

"Lookin' good, Jeremy," they all shout as they enter, greeted in turn, by his big grin.

∼

The day before Jeremy is scheduled to leave rehab, he still uses a metal walker to maneuver, although he can walk alone with a cane at times. The nurses begin to teach him how to use the catheter on his own.

"I need some clothes from my apartment," he informs me on the phone. And I realize this early morning exchange is a contact call, signaling Jeremy's desire to talk about whatever is racing through his mind. He usually chats with Linda, his mother, about such matters. Often up before me, today she is still in bed.

"The nurse did the scan for the catheter around midnight, but didn't fully empty the bladder. So I had to go again around 4:00 AM, but I was half-asleep. So the nurse helped."

Three hours later, Jeremy calls again. Linda, battling her own pain, has gone to see a physical therapist. So I answer, something I almost always avoid now if Linda is home.

"I just walked a long way with the cane," he says, his tone ebullient. "And up and down some stairs, too. I don't need to take a walker home, the therapist said, unless you and Mom feel more comfortable with it."

Jeremy moving from the wheelchair to the metal walker to the cane—our son in motion, making progress: exciting news, I suppose, depending on your perspective. I try to make a joke, echoing what Dr. Groff told Jeremy before he left Beth Israel: "Throw away that cane. We'll walk out of the rehab center together," I say.

"I also feel closer to being able to urinate," Jeremy counters, dodging my attempt at humor.

∼

In his green Allendale Country Club golf shirt and red Bermuda shorts, my neighbor Dennis stands out on the street between our houses and hands me a bottle of holy water from Fatima in Portugal. "Put some on Jeremy's forehead," he insists. He wants to be helpful. Perhaps it will work, along with all the prayers people continue to offer for Jeremy. I don't know; is it possible?

I do know Jeremy got rid of the get-well card from the Rabbi, the card with the Hebrew prayer on it:

Heal us, O Lord, and we shall be healed; save us, and we will be saved, for the one we praise is You. Bring complete healing for all our sicknesses, O God, for You are our faithful and compassionate Healer and King. Blessed are You, Lord, the Healer of the sick of Israel. – Jeremiah 17:14

When his friends came to visit him the other day, Jeremy ripped the card from the corked lined bulletin board on the wall in his hospital room and then threw it in the wastebasket. He refuses to flee into what he insists are signs of false comfort.

I doubt he will accept the holy water without a fuss, either. If I tried to sprinkle the water on his forehead, it would just make him angry. And I'm sure he wouldn't travel with me to Brazil to see John of God, although I continue to consider that bizarre possibility as well.

When I come back in the house with the holy water, Linda has a suggestion: "We should give Jeremy a break. Let's not visit until late afternoon. He'll be stuck with us for a long time after we take him home tomorrow."

We drive over to Wainer's food emporium in New Bedford and shop around for a basket of assorted fruit for the rehab staff. The shelves overflow with luscious goodies. "Look at this… look at that," Linda says, picking one wonderful basket up after another and admiring how fresh and pretty they all look.

"Will you make up a special package for us to take?" Linda finally asks a friendly clerk behind the counter.

"Of course," the woman replies, cheerfully recommending a large straw basket, one brimming with an assortment of ripe peaches, plump pears, juicy plums, bananas and walnuts, all wrapped in cellophane tied with an attractive red bow.

That afternoon, when we carry the colorful basket to the second floor, the rehab staff immediately spots us, opening their arms wide, dancing with gratitude. They are pleased we have taken time to acknowledge their hard work. They quickly arrange the fresh fruit on white plates near the nurses' station. Enjoying the goodies, they beam broadly throughout the rest of the day. Like neighbors, they stroll with us through the long corridors, offering thanks and solicitude.

Settling in his room, I ask Jeremy what most worries him now that he's preparing to leave rehab. He's ranked his concerns in order, giving the unresponsive bladder top priority.

"Well, I suppose if your bladder's made it to the top of the list, you're doing well," I say, another half-witted attempt at humor. "It could've been paralysis, a total disaster, sixty-six percent chance of not walking at all," I remind him—and myself. "And what if Mom and I had already left for our cruise before the paralysis set in?"

"I don't think I can work much either," he responds, disturbed that he might lose the thread of that important part of his identity. "I'll need to relax, watch Netflix. Read a few good books."

"My bank account is modest but secure," he adds after a minute or two. He recently looked up the account on the computer reserved for patients in a small room in the back, the same computer he uses to email his friends and keep them updated, although he seems to prefer text-messaging on his cell phone for that kind of communication.

"And I won't have to prove myself in that swimming match next week down in Maryland," he explains, a competitive match he bet on with his old friends from Tufts before this surprise in his life. They all planned to drive down to Baltimore to watch the Red Sox play at Camden Yard. No pressure for that kind of manly performance right now.

"I'd like to make out a menu for some good meals at your house while I'm there," he also jokes with an ironic smile at the end. He's thinking about his hippie physical therapist, I'm sure.

Like Linda, the doctors and other staff members sound upbeat as we prepare to leave the rehab center. "He's going to be fine," they insist when they gather in his room to wish him well. "Look at him now. See how far he has come." But, for me, and I suspect for Jeremy, the concern about the bladder dangles out there as if on the edge of a dangerous precipice. "I am not worried," the doctor might say. But he is not the one slipping into a vexed future.

In the meantime, I look to the poets—like Wallace Stevens, who helps me understand the strange journey we are all on:

> *I was the world in which I walked, and what I saw*
> *Or heard or felt came not but from myself;*
> *And there I found myself more truly and more strange.*

Walking through the world, we meet ourselves, sometimes as strangers and sometimes as friends, but always ourselves, coming and going.

Our House

Fewer than three weeks have passed since our son was jolted from his ordinary life and thrown across the border. But it seems as if it has been forever.

At home, Linda and I prepare the house for him. We vacuum the rugs, clean the shelves and dust the furniture. Linda puts new sheets on the bed upstairs and fresh towels on the rack in the bathroom. The comfortable brown leather chair we picked out at La-Z-Boy for Jeremy to sit in while taking his antibiotics arrives mid-morning, and then I drive to his apartment to get some of his shorts and tee shirts and a few of his many books.

Jeremy is a deep and rapid reader, and he has already started a reading marathon. He reads a book every three or four days—good books, novels of substance, stories that can break the frozen sea within us, as the writer Franz Kafka once put it.

In his apartment, I examine the novels he has on his shelves, and then rifle through the clothes in his bureau drawers, recalling the time when I traveled to New York to empty Jonathan's lonely apartment after we brought him to Butler Hospital in Providence. He was just beginning his ferocious battle to overcome his addiction then. His cotton knit shirts and Bermuda shorts, his sweaters and towels, even his underwear were all folded so neatly in those bureau drawers in New York; his clothes, so clean and orderly, offered me signs of his struggle against the chaos and dread swirling around him. Like Jeremy now,

Jonathan was so anxious then, lying in his hospital room, wondering if he would ever get better.

When I return home carrying Jeremy's clothes and piles of books, Linda waits near the door. "Jeremy phoned from rehab," she says, beaming. "I could hear the excitement in his voice. He said he was able to urinate a little bit on his own." My muscles relax, untying hard knots deep in my body. But I hold tight against too much hope.

> *"Hope" is the thing with feathers—*
> *That perches in the soul—*
> *And sings the tune without the words—*
> *And never stops—at all—*
> *And sweetest—in the Gale—is heard—*
> *And sore must be the storm—*
> *That could abash the little Bird*
> *That kept so many warm...*   – Emily Dickinson

At the rehab center, we chat briefly with Abramson, thanking him for his care and kindness. "I appreciate your patience and good will," I tell him, while I mindlessly review and sign the various bureaucratic forms for Jeremy's release.

Then a nurse enters the room, helps Jeremy settle in his wheelchair and pushes him down the long corridor. They stop on the way to the elevator to say good-bye to Pete; I rush down the stairs to the parking lot to bring the car around. As I pull up, I see Jeremy sitting outside near the door, Linda and his nurse next to him. He has his cane resting across the arms of the wheelchair, waiting.

Linda and the nurse help Jeremy stand as he takes his cane from the chair. I get out of the driver's seat, hurry around the car and open the right front door. His round face shines with dignity as he slowly walks with his cane to the car and, with effort, slides carefully into the passenger seat next to me. Linda sits exhausted in the back.

For Jeremy, the ride home is a long one, about an hour on the highway. He has not been outside in the summer sun like this—nor has he driven this way in the warm air—for some time. At our house, he flops down on his new leather chair in our living room. He's happy to be out of the institution, back to a house, even if it's not his own. I bring him a pizza without cheese; he is lactose-intolerant. He eats only half of it; the best he can do.

∼

In the suburb of Dartmouth, our house, a free standing condominium with an extensive back porch, looks down into the tree-lined valley below. On the first floor, a master bedroom with connecting bathroom flows into a living room, then a dining room with a long, polished table and comfortable, padded chairs, and finally a kitchen with granite counters. The floors are covered with oriental rugs, the walls with beautiful paintings and lithographs. The living room opens to the second floor, the walls extending up two stories, a balcony overhanging that remarkable sense of space.

A staircase, just to the left of the front door, leads up the stairs to two additional bedrooms. We have converted one bedroom to a study with a marble table and computer, extensive bookcases and an easy chair for reading. The other bedroom is now reserved for Jeremy. The condo is a perfect place for Linda and me, comfortable and aesthetically pleasing. It is our home, giving us symmetry and balance, and we want Jeremy to feel that is his home as well.

Jeremy quickly overcomes his fear of working the rubber catheter by himself. "It's easier to do it alone," he tells us. "Much faster than when I had to wait for the nurse with her full bladder scan." But it is not as easy as he claims.

Long after midnight, upstairs, Jeremy carefully gets out of his king-sized bed and wanders across the wooden floor into the bathroom. His catheter "set-up" is laid out in front of him. The rubber tubing and his bottle to pee-in sit waiting on a clean cotton towel. All of this paraphernalia rests on a frail folding chair that he pulls near the toilet for ease and support when he arrives.

In the bathroom, he flicks on the light switch and quietly closes the door, not wanting to disturb us below.

Suddenly he shouts in a loud voice down to us. It must be 3:00 AM. He stands in his light-blue pajamas, the ten-inch red scar running through his flesh along his spine. "I need some sterile gloves," he bellows from the balcony. "I don't have any on the chair."

We rise from our bed and bring him the gloves. He quietly closes the bathroom door behind him, and we return downstairs to our room. Lying in our bed, we wait until we hear him wandering from the bathroom back across the balcony to his own soft mattress. The next morning he tells us, "I was trying to get your attention for about fifteen minutes before you responded."

Thank goodness he didn't give up.

~

Emma, one of Jeremy's community nurses, comes to the house to help with the intravenous infusion early in the morning and again in the evening when the sun sets.

The physical therapist, Kelly, calls: "I'll be over tomorrow morning at 11:00 or 11:15," she says. Jeremy reads and watches television in his new brown leather chair in our living room. The soft texture of the Barcalounger soothes his body when he sits in it. He floats and dreams when he settles there.

Robert Sawyer, his primary care physician, phones late in the afternoon to hear the details of Jeremy's story. He is a compassionate and caring man, and we count on the doctor to serve as an anchor and advocate if the situation dictates.

Listening to Jeremy talk to Dr. Sawyer, I hear the same story he told yesterday at our house to the lead nurse, an administrative veteran. She was getting everything in order for the long month ahead. We sat on the cushioned chairs then, talking across the room as she reviewed his case, asking a series of questions for the record.

"I'm much better now," Jeremy insisted. "Much better."

He's making it up, I thought. He's trying to sound as if he were all but cured. "Jeremy, that's not quite true," I said to him and to the head nurse. I didn't want her recording inaccurate information.

The nurse was good about it. Her neck bent over her clipboard, she shook her head with understanding. "Yes, I actually had all this information down in my notes long before Jeremy said anything," she replied with a reassuring tone, a sign of her efficiency.

Jeremy was displaying his peacock feathers, his pride and courage, but he wasn't describing the reality, and she clearly knew that.

I don't want Dr. Sawyer to misunderstand now, over the phone with Jeremy.

"You've been through hell and back," Sawyer tells him. The doctor believes that Jeremy has already returned from hell. I don't think Jeremy has. I don't want Sawyer to think so either.

Many people care about Jeremy, but they offer false analogies for his pain—defense strategies to keep their own locations close and secure. "Oh, it's like the time I had a terrible backache," they say; or, "Oh, my brother had to have a bacterial infection cleaned from his discs once"; or, "Oh, I had back surgery a couple of times. That's tough"; or, "Oh, I had to use a catheter for two weeks myself after leaving the hospital once."

We prefer to stay on this side of the border, the invisible line that keeps us hidden from ourselves.

After Jonathan's death, even good friends believed Linda and I had a disease. If they came too close to us, they'd catch that sickness. We were contagious, carriers of rotting flesh. How often Linda came home from the supermarket, her body bursting with anger or her face streaming with tears. "I can't believe it," she would say. "I saw our neighbor today standing at the corner of the aisle, and she turned around so quickly I thought she'd twist her ankle trying to avoid me. She didn't think I saw her when she bolted in the opposite direction."

∼

Our house is turning into a Salvador Dali painting: bizarre machinery and wires connected to human body parts; strange digital contraptions flickering and humming next to ordinary kitchen appliances; colorless prescription drugs placed on refrigerator shelves close to red tomatoes and crispy green celery stalks.

Linda works side by side with Jeremy to manage the new gadgets and medical equipment. They slowly master the most difficult challenge: setting up the intravenous infusion twice a day. The process in the evening is more complicated than the one in the morning. In both cases, they push the antibiotics from a small bag through a needle into his right arm, then they set a larger bag dripping from the pole through the intravenous line. In the evening, before the infusion begins, the line itself needs to be changed and threaded through the pump machine, made ready for the PICC line in his arm.

An automated monitor blinks in the kitchen, measuring Jeremy's blood pressure, oxygen levels, heart rate and body weight. The small contraption sits on a shelf, close to the coffee maker and the shiny metal toaster.

The monitor is connected through the phone wires to the central health office across the river in Fairhaven. Like a cyborg, Jeremy sends the data through the monitor at around 10:30 each morning; then someone at the office reads the results and calls a few minutes later if there is anything odd to report.

Up early Sunday morning, I go to buy some whitefish, bagels, chopped liver, lox and cream cheese at the deli down the street while Jeremy, without nursing assistance, runs his intravenous drip. When I come in the door, he has a wide grin on his weary face as he sits patiently in his leather chair. He is hungry.

Later we notice a rash developing on his arms and a high heart rate on the pulse monitor—around 120.

∽

"Dad," Jeremy asks, "do you think my nurse Emma is so kind and considerate because she is Jewish?" Emma, a small and thin woman, with light brown hair and wire-rimmed glasses, emigrated from Russia because of the mistreatment of Jews there. She has extended herself for us. "You'll be able to run that IV infusion yourself. Believe me; don't worry," she said when she first came to the house. And that gave us confidence. "I know how difficult this is for all of you," she empathized, her eyes glazed over with tears when we told her about Jonathan. "It will work out this time, I know," she promised. And that gave us comfort. "I only live a few blocks from here," she explained. "Call me anytime." And we did.

Jeremy might have a point about this fragile woman; her suffering has not hardened her to the brute facts but graced her with compassion. Emma stands out.

"Emma reminds me of Emmanuel Levinas, a French thinker who developed a theory of ethical vulnerability," I say to Jeremy.

"Oh, really, Dad," Jeremy responds, uncertain if he wants to hear this.

"Levinas believes that the person standing before us is always to be considered first, as if that person is always more important than we are," I tell Jeremy. "Pay careful attention to 'the face' of the person in front of us, Levinas suggests. Be a witness."

Jeremy grins at me. "Here I am, Dad," he says.

"That is the ethical demand for Levinas. Pay careful attention to the person before you."

"Sounds right to me." Jeremy says in agreement.

"But not everyone would agree," I remind him. "Some might consider such behavior foolish. Makes you an easy target, a *schlemiel*."

"Like the characters from Yiddish literature—Singer's Gimpel the Fool or Peretz's Bontsha the Silent?" Jeremy responds.

"Right. Those saintly fools get a bad rap these days. They're not sluggers. Remember what Gimpel says? 'I am Gimpel the Fool. I don't think myself a fool. On the contrary. But that's what folks call me.'"

I look directly at Jeremy, and continue: "The students always tell me, 'This guy should get tough. Be more assertive. Learn to cope. Suck it up. Stand up like a man. Be strong.'"

"Maybe Levinas is a little like Gandhi or King," Jeremy concludes. "Passive resistance."

∼

Jeremy anticipates his first acupuncture treatment with my childhood friend, Danny Schwartz, whose red hair and open manner earn him well deserved recognition as a sensitive and fiery healer. When the visiting nurse arrives early in the morning, though, she checks Jeremy's intravenous lines and discovers a tiny puncture. It needs immediate attention, given the ongoing demand to pump the crucial antibiotics through the line twice a day, on schedule, into Jeremy's bloodstream.

"We'll have to get this fixed ASAP," the nurse says, surprised that I'm calling Beth Israel before she's finished talking.

The hospital staff respond quickly: "Bring Jeremy to the day clinic in the Farr Building around noon."

Beth Israel is phantom territory for us; we'd prefer not to go back so quickly, but what choice do we have? Reluctantly, I cancel Jeremy's acupuncture appointment, and we're off.

On the road, Jeremy sits next to me, listening to Mahler's Second Symphony on the radio. It's an hour drive, and he tries endlessly to adjust his anxious body. The music transports him; the rough leather on the seats irritates his spine. Behind him, in the back of the car, Linda fidgets. She stares out the side window, her head throbbing from the oppressive heat. Dark sunglasses hide her eyes while she flips the air conditioning vent up and down.

When we pull up in front of the Farr Building, Jeremy slides carefully from his seat onto the pavement. He is wobbly, but relieved just to stand up. Linda helps him across the sidewalk into the hospital. By the time I return from the parking lot, they're waiting for the nurse practitioner to summon us in for the procedure.

"This'll be easy," the nurse claims. She draws out the old PICC and inserts a new one through his hand and up into his right arm. Although cautious, she twice pushes the new line through his neck rather than down toward his heart. After the second attempt, we're all frustrated and on edge. "I'm sorry," she says. "I thought we could do this procedure down here, but I'm going to send Jeremy upstairs to the radiology department. Perhaps they'll have more luck guided by x-ray technology."

Unfortunately, the radiology team encounters its own troubles. A difficult procedure for Jeremy, he lies quietly without anesthesia or painkillers, while the team watches the x-ray screen hanging from the ceiling. They work very slowly, chatting to each other about their plans for the upcoming weekend. They poke and prod, push and pull. Eventually they position the PICC line through his arm and down near his heart. The plastic tubing is finally back inside his body.

Linda and I read old magazines in a cramped waiting area down the corridor for much longer than we expected. When they wheel Jeremy out of the x-ray room, I see the PICC line inserted in his hand, dry blood caking all around the entry point.

"Looks like you had some problems there," I say annoyed with the team in their white professional uniforms.

"No, we didn't," they claim. "What you're seeing is normal."

"They kept saying how 'weird' all this was," Jeremy tells me later. "As if there were something wrong."

Language deserves our care, I think. We need more than diagnosis and technical procedures.

I push Jeremy in his metal wheelchair through the white pipe-lined basement tunnel of the hospital, whizzing through that capsule-like space, picking up speed and laughing as we go. Linda runs next to us. We are beneath the street, heading over to the Infectious Disease Clinic to check the rash on his skin.

Jeremy is weary, but Linda wants to see if the medical team can provide some remedy for him. Anxious for small victories, she's trying to be optimistic and practical. Unfortunately, the doctors offer no explanation for his rash.

~

Jeremy's cane thumps against the wooden planks above me. It's as if I'm Ishmael in my bunk listening to Ahab's peg leg stumping across the deck of Herman Melville's fictional whaleship, the *Pequod*. Early Sunday morning, Jeremy again makes that lonely journey across our wooden balcony, headed to that place of silence where all his paraphernalia waits for him.

Sensing Jeremy's movement upstairs, I doze off, dreaming about Jonathan: how Jonathan loved to race across the soft rugs in our old apartment, so many years ago, when he was still a young boy; his loud laughter echoing through the room as he threw wide the cabinets at the edge of the living room carpet; his hands, a blur in endless motion, knocking objects from the shelves; small painted vases rolling across the rug; his laughter like a silver sparkler, flaming for an instant, crackling through the dense air, quickly fading into the darkness.

Tomorrow, August 20, marks the twelfth anniversary of Jonathan's death. Like Jeremy's, Jonathan's astonishing journey into the vortex of bitter night startled us. Palpable memories of detox centers and halfway houses, blood infections and hospital beds evoke new nightmares now as I toss and turn, wrapped in the suffocating air.

In one nightmare, stars glitter on my body and then, like tears, they fall from my flesh, dripping to the hard ground turning to mud at my feet. The image, a fragment disturbing time, stirs other dreams screaming through my rebellious body.

At dawn, my hands clasped behind my head, eyes fixed on the white ceiling, Jonathan's voice whispers from the walls: "Are you there, Dad? Are you there?" His voice, twisting round and round in my ears, throws me further off balance.

In the daylight, Linda and I go outdoors. The bright sun splashes across the green grass. Linda points to a small branch of lilies, her mother's favorite flower, blooming near the side of our house. Ordinarily these flowers only bloom at the beginning of spring, then not again until the following year. "It's a sign that Jonathan is looking over Jeremy," she says with warmth and certainty. "And my mother is watching him, too."

But the rosebush near our back porch, rooted to Jonathan's memory, has yet to blossom this year. "That's a sign Jonathan is spending all his energy helping to heal Jeremy," Linda says. "And notice the green leaves flourishing on the rosebush," she adds. "So it's just a matter of time before Jeremy returns to full bloom."

The softness and the poetry in the cadence and flow of her words soothe my troubled flesh. But, as I listen, other words brush through me—like the description of the young Euphorbus's death in Homer's *Iliad*, a moment of harsh winds uprooting even the strongest of earthly vines:

> *Imagine the hearty shoot of an olive which a man cultivates in a lonely place and generously waters, and it blooms beautifully. And the breaths of all the winds cause it to tremble, and pale flowers burst forth from it. Then suddenly a storm comes up with mighty blasts and rips it from the ground and lays it flat. So it was with Euphorbus, the son of Panthus, when Menelaus killed him and stripped his armor off.* – trans. by David Gill, SJ

I will not sleep well tonight.

At sunset, the three of us seek out the synagogue to recite the mourner's prayer, Kaddish, for Jonathan. There are just ten people at the service, a *minyan*; only one knows what has happened to Jeremy. Our son sits quietly next to us, a Hebrew prayer book in his hands. He cannot stand up, a custom for the recitation of some of the prayers, but he has insisted on joining us tonight to pay respect to his brother. Perhaps I should develop more community support for Jeremy as I did for Jonathan, I think.

And suddenly, in the midst of that small gathering, I feel a tug. Concealed, behind the beautifully carved wooden doors of the holy ark, the Torah scrolls sing. I cannot see those ancient scrolls, but I sense their presence beckoning to me. The Hebrew letters dance on the parchment; I am wrapped in awe.

In the synagogue, the tiny congregation rapidly chants the evening service, the sun sets outside, and dusk creeps across the windows. The hard benches trouble Jeremy's back. He holds his body tight, feeling the spasms radiate through his legs, as we complete the mourner's prayer.

When the three of us leave the small sanctuary, all the roads seem empty. The orange moon haunts the gray sky. We go straight home so Jeremy can take some pain medication.

~

Jeremy loves books. Since his operation, he will have read almost fifty novels before the new year. They include:

Seize the Day	*Falling Man*	*Another Bullshit Night*
The Book of Ralph	*LA Rex*	*in Sick City*
The Child in Time	*Amsterdam*	*Things My Girlfriend and*
Never Let Me Go	*Company*	*I Have Argued About*
Black Swan Green	*Child of God*	*Wherever You Go, There*
Man Gone Down	*The Defense*	*You Are*
On Chesil Beach	*The Natural*	*Extremely Loud and*
Yiddish Detectives	*Dopefiend*	*Incredibly Close*
Fortunate Son	*Disgrace*	*The Comfort of Strangers*
The Cement Garden	*Neon Bible*	*Waiting for the Barbarians*
A Black Girl Lost	*Last One In*	*My Legendary Girlfriend*
The Book of Daniel	*The Big Sleep*	*In the Heart of the Country*
Crossing California	*The Road*	*The Abstinence Teacher*
The Ginger Man	*Last Night*	*How to Talk to a Widower*
The Southpaw	*Rabbit Run*	*The New York Trilogy*
The Alchemist	*Black Dogs*	*A Certain Chemistry*

Like medicine on a shelf, these books need to be taken in and digested by a sensitive reader, and Jeremy is just that kind of reader, the kind that lets language seep deep through the skin and permeate the heart. Such reading gives him buoyancy, a lightness of being. Good books stir his blood and transport him to some other place.

But Jeremy is weighted down by that other medicine: antibiotics through the intravenous drip, four hours each day; Vancomycin and

Roseferin kept chilled on the bottom shelf of the refrigerator, not far from the butter and the milk; Zoloft for anxiety; Hydrochlorothiazide and Atenelol for blood pressure; Hydrocodone and Advil for pain; Urecholine for the bladder; Colace for stool softening; Pepsid for stomach acid.

And his liver enzymes are slightly elevated. I wonder how they could be otherwise, given all these pharmaceuticals pulsating through his blood stream.

∽

When our children look at our face, they gaze into a mirror. It does not matter how young or old they are. They could be three or thirty or twice that. Our heartbeat is bound to theirs. The flow of their blood runs through our veins, and our blood runs through theirs.

Linda tries to be optimistic for this reason. She has vowed to be so. She wants to mirror hope for Jeremy, and in the process, she protects herself, clothed with the richly woven colors that allow for boundaries and distance. She is practical and reasonable.

We must celebrate small victories won as we walk along this difficult valley, she says.

She makes a list for practical guidance and instruction:

1. Keep Jeremy content and comfortable.
2. Prepare his environment so he can do his work of regeneration and make his bid for independence.
3. Cheer Jeremy on.

But just beneath the skin, Jeremy is distressed, and I find such lists insufficient for such heartache.

Our son is at times enraged, at times frustrated, at times depressed. Sometimes he is silent, feeling he must hide from the world swirling around him. Sometimes he's ready to shout, his life like a swelling tumult rising to a shattering explosion.

∽

Caught in a whirlwind, spinning from doctor to doctor, we make our way up Route 140, past the Silver City Galleria, and then over to Route 24, sweeping quickly by the Burger King in Bridgewater and the ramshackled mall in Brockton, headed to Beth Israel again—this time to see the neurosurgeon.

"Try not to move," a medical technician instructs Jeremy as she fits him snugly into the MRI capsule, his eyes closed, music streaming through the ear plugs attached to his iPod. Squeezed tight in that capsule, his back pounds for nearly an hour. He wishes he could fly with the astronauts to the moon. Finally, he's out of the machine, and we wheel him through the underground tunnel to Dr. Groff's office for an update on his progress.

"I forgot to bring my kit," Jeremy tells me when we get to the office; I wander over to the triage area to pick up a straight catheter for him, while he sits with Linda in the waiting room. It's only noon, and he's already spent, bent over from the long day.

When the nurse calls his name, though, Jeremy jumps up from his chair, greeting the doctor with an energetic handshake. He's determined to show Dr. Groff how well he is doing. No doubt Groff is an excellent surgeon, sharp and well focused, but he's not someone who enjoys discussions with patients. We need to realize that, as he ushers us to a small room in his suite of inner offices.

The doctor examines Jeremy carefully, first checking his back and then pushing against his legs to test how well those legs resist pressure. He nods as he moves his agile hands across his patient's body, clearly impressed by the progress. I watch Groff closely, recalling when Dr. Shen raised Jeremy's leg from the gurney that first night, and we saw that leg drop, falling like lead to the grimed ground.

When asked, Groff says he sees no residual effect from the surgery. Good news. He's proud of his work. We're all pleased.

"But what about the future?" I ask Groff, who seems pressed, the physical examination complete. "Should we take Jeremy to a neurourologist? You realize, I imagine, his bladder still doesn't work right."

Dr. Groff rejects my suggestion. "Let the body heal on its own. They can't do anything right now anyway," he points out. "No reason to take Jeremy anywhere else, as long as he makes steady improvement."

"Makes steady improvement"? I'm not sure what that phrase means in this context, but I let the remark slide.

Then Groff startles us: "Jeremy can now do whatever he's capable of. Drive a car if he wants to. Return to work."

"No need for further physical therapy," the doctor adds, speaking directly to Jeremy. "Exercise on your own when you feel like it, after another week or so."

He's talking too fast, but I remain quiet. Jeremy appears bewildered. Linda stands to the side, intent on Groff. She too appears puzzled, but satisfied with the report. Apparently she's keeping her fierce mother love in tight check.

The only restriction for Jeremy now is to avoid heavy lifting: "Nothing above fifty pounds." Other than that, he should listen to what his body tells him and act accordingly.

Trust your body when that body has betrayed you? That sounds like a contradiction to me. And to leave Jeremy right now with so little structure and no clear medical plan appears outrageous, as if a rug has suddenly been pulled from under him, setting him spinning.

What is Groff thinking about? I'd like to know. We leave the upstairs office and the doctor departs in the other direction to prepare for his scheduled afternoon surgery. Perhaps Groff is purposely taking a positive and activist stance here. But I am concerned. Jeremy needs firmer direction, a better-defined context to deal with his pain.

Out in the busy Boston streets, Jeremy drifts ahead of us. He's gathering his thoughts, but beneath his sweating skin there's obvious distress. "Should I go back to work on Monday?" he asks. "What shall I tell my friends?" he wonders. "They'll all expect me to go out with them; what shall I do?"

Groff has acknowledged Jeremy's suffering, how difficult this ordeal has been for him, how tired Jeremy must be. But the surgeon is already focused on his next operation. By contrast, we are scattered, out in open space, breathing the turbulent city air humming around us.

While we roam the sidewalks, I picture Jeremy with his friends on New Year's Eve this past year. Four good friends, traveling down to Rio to party hard on the beaches—Copacabana, Ipanema. Millions of young and energetic bodies sparkle in that Dionysian rapture, shouting and celebrating the birth of the new year. They fly high and free while the ocean roars in the wild, erotic splendor of sand and surf. There he is, our son, in all his raucous glory, watching colorful fireworks explode like lightning in the night sky. Only a few months ago.

Jeremy's body refuses to function well the rest of the day, as we all stumble down the crowded Boston streets on this late August afternoon, listening to the taxis blowing their horns, the cars whistling by. Eventually we get in our own car and travel slowly out of the bustling city and back home to Dartmouth.

∾

Armies of medical professionals have stabbed Jeremy's body, invaded its territory. They have subjugated it and tried to redefine it. They offer endless opinions. But separate from all medical intervention, the body has its own flow, its own secret language. Perhaps this is what Groff meant. Listen to your own body; it speaks to you from the secret recesses of its own knowledge.

I want all those secrets to be articulated, all concealment revealed. I want to hear the heart beating, the legs shouting with vitality, the bones whispering with a strong flourish, the back upright with straight talk. And I want the bladder to shout out to us, gushing like a cow at full force in a sunny meadow, soft and sweet.

I have heard Jeremy's body speak to us already, say to us what was unknown, silent, but there. I have seen the movement of his legs after paralysis give all of us new breath, his back bellow with joy as he stood for the first time near his hospital bed. I have listened to his bones and nerves, his muscles and sinews awakening beneath his skin as he walked.

We hope for the full articulation of that body now. We insist on it. It is what Jeremy yearns for, what we all demand.

Like the buds of a flower, the future unfolds through our children, and, if we are fortunate, we find aesthetic beauty in that process, hope and justice, dreams as well.

I, however, find no adequate compensation for Jonathan's death, no just balance for that absence. Jonathan lives only as a ghost in my memory, as words in a book, as laughter heard in a silent room. Turning to dust in the tomb, his bones haunt me. No aesthetic beauty, no memories from the grave compensate for the ugliness of loss, especially the loss of a child. Such violent loss evokes a covenant broken, a promise betrayed. Jonathan lives now only through the memory of his story, a revenant rustling through the bones of all those who care to remember him.

Jeremy shakes me to the bone, too. With Jonathan, he stirs in my flesh. It is as if grief has been stitched twice through my body. When I look at Jeremy's troubled eyes and his pale skin, I see his longing and I see Jonathan's as well. Their aching hearts beat on my pulse. I know that my glance, at such moments, rattles Jeremy. He does not want to be the cause of my pain, and I only want to heal his. That I cannot heal him is my agony.

Some say, I am obsessed.

∼

Jeremy continues his rigorous exercise with Kelly, the physical therapist, inside our house and outside, along the driveway and walkways, in the late-summer air. Kelly, young and tall, blonde and athletic, pushes Jeremy to his limit. She watches him inside the house when he struggles up and down the steep stairs and when he lies on his soft bed, raising and lowering his legs. She strolls with him outside, up and down the driveway, over the paths, across the hills of the black-tarred road. Resting the full weight of his spent body on his sturdy cane, he catches his breath, while the curls of his light brown hair sparkle like diamonds caressed by the summer breeze.

Jeremy works with his acupuncturist, Danny, as well. Clearly the acupuncturist wishes him good health. Danny is a caring man and seasoned professional, serving Jeremy over several sessions now.

One day in his office, Indian music plays in the background, while incense permeates the sweet air. Danny, frustrated, looks at Jeremy stretched out on the table and says: "You seem to be stagnating." The phrase startles Jeremy, just as his friends rattled him this morning on the phone when they jokingly suggested with their own style of masculine gusto: "Maybe you'll never be able to piss again." Stunned by his buddies, Jeremy could only reply, "That's not really very funny. I'm making progress, you know."

Jeremy's friends care, but language can penetrate the skin like a sharp pin, deflate us like a punctured balloon, and stir up infection much like the instruments of a neurosurgeon. We cannot afford to be careless.

Danny cares, too. "There's a connection between the feet and the kidneys running up through the back," he suggests. He wants to break through the "stagnation" by stimulating the networks of communication. Set Jeremy free. Open the flood gates. Let him saunter.

"I'm going to burn the soles of your feet," the red-haired acupuncturist says. Jeremy squirms on the table. The burning of the soles of the feet is an ancient Chinese procedure employed to excite the flow of the body. Jeremy agrees to it, and endures the fire, despite discomfort, believing that, yes, perhaps it will help. It's worth a try.

The poet Marge Piercy put it this way:

> *We stand in the midst of the burning world*
> *primed to burn with compassionate love and justice,*
> *to turn inward and find holy fire at the core,*
> *to turn outward and see the world that is all*
> *of one flesh with us…*

∽

For over a month, Jeremy has made certain that no bubbles form when his medicine drips through the plastic tubing attached to the pole near his chair, down into his battered arm, then through his body. He can't wait to return to his own apartment. Today he's excited, anticipating that Dr. Gardner at the Infectious Disease Clinic will announce he's disease-free and can take his PICC line out.

Gardner's waiting room overflows with patients, many with AIDS. Some sit by themselves. Some look like skeletons, barely able to walk. While we wait for almost three hours, the Buddhist Thich Nhat Hanh's words dance through the room: "People usually consider walking on water or in thin air a miracle. But I think the real miracle is not to walk either on water or in thin air, but to walk on earth." Earth walkers, I imagine. We are all earth walkers here.

Finally, we're called.

About the same age as Jeremy, thirty-two or thirty-three years old, Gardner looks like Doogie Houser, the young doctor with a Howdy Doodie face from the television show a few years ago. Gardner has already worked a long and hectic morning, but he stands healthy next to Jeremy, who slumps slightly as he leans forward on the edge of the examination table. The doctor glances at the chart on his clipboard, and reiterates what we have heard from Groff: "The MRI shows no signs of infection or traces of bacteria on the bone." Jeremy's liver enzymes remain moderately high, but Dr. Gardner is not particularly concerned; he'll run some additional blood tests as a precaution.

"You should finish the intravenous infusion on Friday night," he announces, words greeted with a gust of joy and then calm relief. "Saturday is officially the end of the six weeks."

"Do we have any statistics giving us odds for relapse?"

"No formal studies, but the odds are probably not much different for Jeremy than for anyone else."

Then Gardner offers up another one of those piercing phrases: "You'll soon face 'the critical period,'" he says, "the period after the antibiotics are finished." The critical period, yes, the critical period when Jeremy will be first exposed to the capacious world beyond our house. Out in open space, Jeremy will no longer have the luxury of medical protection running through his bloodstream.

Finally I ask Dr. Gardner the inevitable question, the nagging one that frustrates Jeremy whenever he hears it, the one that mirrors back his own agony: "What about the nerve regeneration; what about the bladder?"

And Gardner offers the usual response: "Little can be done, other than to wait. It all depends on the healing of the spinal cord, which still has some swelling."

∼

Like a bright sturgeon moon—the kind that the astronauts perhaps envisioned in 1969—Jeremy's face beams with pleasure, anticipating the upcoming weekend. On Saturday, he will be untangled from the medical machinery, from the wires and meddling, from the annoying confinement and restriction he's endured at our house. Moving around his apartment on his own, Jeremy thinks he'll be free to roam the sky. But such relief represents just a small step, a passing glimpse, reflecting his longing. He will need a giant leap across cratered terrain before he is whole again.

When he first walked up and down the stairs with his physical therapist, her tye-dye charm cheering him on in the Cape Cod rehab center, he staggered then, wobbly with each step. But despite his unsteadiness, he was proud. In motion on those stairs he gazed far beyond the walls of the rehab center. He traveled on the curve of time, eyes fixed to the horizon. Something called to him then, something cloaked in the sun on a hill, something at a distance.

The poet Rilke describes it:

>   *Already my gaze is upon the hill, the sunny one,*
>   *At the end of the path which I've only just begun.*

So we are grasped by that which we could not grasp,
At such great distance, so fully manifest.

And now Jeremy continues to imagine; he envisions his apartment, his freedom, his independence—a new morning. "I've only just begun," he declares.

Jeremy exchanges email and text messages with all his friends across the electronic screens announcing the good news ("free at last, free at last"), and we begin to move his clothing and other possessions back to his apartment. Early tomorrow, his PICC line will be drawn out of his body; that thin tubing, lodged in his right arm and shoved close to his heart for six weeks, will be gone. He will settle in at his apartment, watch movies on his new Blu-ray DVD player, and read long into the night. He will be angry at times, defensive, frustrated and hurt. But he will be drawn forward, seeking to touch the hem of the garment stretching up from the bright earth before him.

"I've been dreaming a lot," he tells me. "In one dream, I go for a job interview at the D.A.'s office, but I have to sit by myself for a long time in the waiting room on a narrow folding chair. It's a huge room, and no one else is there. I feel an urge to go to the bathroom while I wait, but I've forgotten my catheter." He sits in the D.A.'s office, growing angry at me, until the dream fades out.

"I was upset with you, Dad," he says. As his father, I understand, thanks to poet Anthony Hecht who explained it this way to his own son:

Adam, there will be
Many hard hours,
As an old poem says,
Hours of loneliness.
I cannot ease them for you;
They are our common lot.
During them, like as not,
You will dream of me.

Linda would like someone to pick up the intravenous equipment late Saturday afternoon before we get too far into the long Labor Day weekend. She wants that equipment out of our home immediately and forever. But no one from the community pharmacy can manage to come to our house until the following week. Late Saturday night, after Jeremy is done with them for good, I tuck the machine and the pole away, out of sight, in a dusty corner in the garage.

His Apartment

At ease in open space, Jeremy floats free from any sudden doubt, from any quick pull that might ground him. He is back in his own apartment. Sure footed, I walk with pride, as I did when Jonathan and Jeremy left home to become freshmen at college, glimpsing their newly discovered independence, but with hesitation as well, thinking about how they were alone and exposed when the evening light came into their dorm room. My sons felt otherwise, of course, bound in a different direction.

Now Jeremy sleeps soundly in his own king-sized bed, his body wrapped in a frail blanket and clean white sheets. It's the first time in over a month that he's settled there, the first time since we took him from that same bed to the local hospital in late July.

Early Sunday morning, I bring him the *Boston Globe*, some laundry detergent and a new heating pad. He needs to monitor his temperature and blood pressure, so I have brought along two digital thermometers and the kit that I usually use to measure my own heart rhythm and pressure. When I leave, Jeremy looks at peace with himself.

Around noon, Linda and I make our way to OfficeMax to buy Jeremy a new bookcase for the novels spilling over throughout his apartment. It's Labor Day weekend and all the salespeople are busy chatting with other customers, as we inspect the shiny printers and smooth metal desks piled high throughout the store. College students crowd the aisles, shopping for the new semester. Young parents wheel their babies in strollers, seeking holiday bargains. Finally we choose a bookcase that should fit nicely against the wall in Jeremy's spare bedroom, but we can't get anyone to assemble it before we put it in the car.

"Leave it in the cardboard box," Linda insists. "One of his friends will help with the shelves when they come over to visit."

Leave the unopened box in his apartment? Won't Jeremy try to assemble the bookcase himself? Struggling to fit all the pieces together, he'll strain his body, hurt his back. I bring the shelves home and, with my good neighbor Dennis, I assemble the bookcase in the garage.

When I drive back to his apartment complex later in the day, the hot sun seems blistering, the stagnant air stifling. I examine the grounds around the place like a watchdog, checking for any sign of a problem. This is, after all, "the critical period" for my son. Dr. Gardner had said just that.

Jeremy greets me at the door, then staggers over to the couch. I carry the bookcase across the living room and begin to arrange his novels on the empty shelves. Watching me from the couch, Jeremy shakes his head in disbelief: "I can do that."

I spot a small garbage container near his sink. "Okay, I'm leaving," I tell him. "But please don't take that garbage out by yourself. Did you see all the trash piled high near the big bins?—all kinds of flies and bees buzzing around out there on this holiday weekend."

"I promise I won't. I'll ask my friends when they come over later. They'll carry the bags out," he says, as I depart for home.

The following day, Linda, knotted in pain, makes an appointment to see her massage therapist, and Jeremy and I go for lunch at Rosie's, a favorite old restaurant haunt of ours, just a couple of miles from our house. Only a few people are seated at the tables when we walk in. The place seems a lot dirtier than I remembered. The rugs look threadbare. Dust rests in the corners, but we sit down on the straight wooden chairs and order: iced tea for me, diet coke for him, and sandwiches.

Jeremy appears stiff, his spine aching, his legs cramped with spasms. His style is laid back, though, almost too calm. He surveys the familiar room, concerned about how his summer has slipped by so quickly. When I mention the recent confusion about his prescriptions at CVS, he simply shrugs his shoulders. "Big deal," he says. "I'll pick 'em up tomorrow."

The waitress is inordinately slow, and does not come by our table to offer refills on the iced tea and soda. I call another waitress over. "We need some help here," I say sternly, pointing at the empty glasses on the table. "Refills?"

Jeremy is nonchalant about all of it, wondering why I can't show more patience.

"You worry too much," he claims.

But when we get the drinks, he lifts his glass, and with silent approval, nods to me across the table.

∼

"Looks like my spine will be a long-term project," Jeremy announces when we phone to see how his physical therapy went at the Faunce Corner Health Club.

"I was surprised by the exercise bike," he says. Before his surgery in July, he easily spent a solid forty minutes on that bike. Sweating hard, he pumped the pedals with such rapid speed that the spinning wheels almost flew off the frame.

Now everything has changed.

"I could only stay on the seat for six minutes; then my legs got tired," Jeremy tells me.

"Six minutes," I respond, wondering why Dr. Groff didn't insist on additional therapy. "That's pretty good. A lot of people couldn't pedal like that for more than one minute."

"And the therapist recommended new exercises to strengthen my body at home," Jeremy adds, another acknowledgment of the considerable distance he still needs to travel.

"This seems so drawn out. My life is passing me by," he sighs, just before he hangs up the phone and goes into his bedroom to rest.

Later in the week, his voice projects a different tone. We all lunch together in a small Lebanese restaurant half hidden in a strip mall near our house. "I'm peeing much more now," he offers excitedly, glancing up from the table, first with expectation on his face, and then with disappointment.

"Don't you believe me?" he finally asks, uncertain why we're not more enthusiastic about his report.

"Of course, we believe you," we tell him. But we remain cautious, recalling the bags full of urine emptied from his bladder that first night back in July at Beth Israel. How lucky it didn't back up into his kidneys then!

"Why didn't you say something when you couldn't go all that time?" Linda asks, wiping her brow.

"I don't know how it's possible, really. How could anyone not go for almost three days?" Jeremy wonders, his focus drifting from us to a young college girl at the next table, while he eats his Mideast *shwarma* sandwich, his fingers dripping with sauce.

∽

Wednesday, at sunset, the three of us celebrate Rosh Hashana around the round glass table in our kitchen. We light the holiday candles, recite the traditional prayers over the bread and wine, and then feast on scrumptious rib roast with baked potato.

Ordinarily we'd invite our extended family to the house for the evening ritual—my elderly mother and brother, his wife and three children—and we'd all gather around the big polished table in the dining room. I'd distribute small sheets of paper, and each family member would write one wish for the upcoming year. Then we'd each place that wish in a sealed envelope, to be revealed next year around the same table. We'd laugh together, tell family stories and insist that the younger generation, despite their objections, attend the religious service in the morning.

Not tonight. Jeremy cannot sit for long; he won't be with us in the synagogue this Jewish New Year.

At services on Thursday morning, worshippers ask about Jeremy, offering solace. "How is he doing?" they want to know. "I heard he's making good progress," they say. "He's such a fine young man," they agree.

The synagogue is not crowded, at least compared to the old days when Jonathan and Jeremy attended Hebrew School there, singing Jewish melodies to the congregation with their classmates from the *bima* on the High Holidays. Now only a handful of children are left, remnants of the past. Many young families have moved away, seeking opportunity elsewhere.

When we leave the synagogue at the end of the long morning service, we shake hands with other congregants. "L'shana Tova," we say, wishing everyone the best for the new year.

I agree to go to the Providence Place mall after the synagogue services on Friday, the second day of the holiday. Jeremy maps out the trip for me.

"You and I can browse in the bookstore first, while Mom goes up to Nordstrom. Then we'll go to the Cheesecake Factory for lunch and finally over to Whole Foods for weekend supplies. I'd like to get back in time for the Yankee game—okay, Dad?" he asks.

Jeremy likes to end conversations with an agreeable question. He rarely wears sharp edges, clothing himself in indirection, whether in court or with friends and family. He's sensitive and determined but not overly aggressive.

When he served as an assistant district attorney, he cross-examined a retired judge in the Attleboro courtroom once. The judge's friend was accused of driving to a high school football game with open beer cans in his car. "Be diplomatic and respectful to that witness," Jeremy had been warned. Fair enough, he thought; I'll circle, but not pounce. I don't want to be disagreeable, but I need to make sure justice stands out.

At the crucial moment, Jeremy leaned in. The courtroom was crowded; the retired judge was testifying on the stand. "With all due respect, sir," Jeremy began, "you, as a judge, must have known—didn't you?—when you were driving up to the stadium with your good friend, that there shouldn't be any open cans in the car." You could hear the hush in the halls of justice then, the scales of justice straining for balance, and then the click, those scales settling into place. Win or lose, Jeremy had made his point with honor and dignity. Justice had spoken, and everyone in the courthouse knew it.

As soon as the trial was over, all the court officials rushed up to Jeremy and shook his hand. "High fives all around," they shouted, laughing with recognition. "You've got balls, I'll tell you that," they exclaimed, as Jeremy with his head held high walked out the front door. He was flying.

Jeremy is a subdued fighter, a man of principle, and we should never underestimate him. Yet now, I can't understand exactly what he needs at times, what he feels beneath the skin. Perhaps he can't either.

"I don't think my bladder fully empties when I use the catheter," he says. I don't challenge his observation, but doubt he's right. What is he really trying to tell me? He circles around points, at times, and refuses to land.

∼

"And they heard the voice of the Lord God walking in the garden in the cool of the day; and Adam and his wife hid themselves from the presence of the Lord God amongst the trees of the garden," the Biblical text says.

My Jewish literature class sits in front of me in their wooden chairs. "We hide our faces because we do not want to see the faces of others," I tell my students. They look up at me, but they seem bored; they prefer reading the Yiddish stories, "Gimpel the Fool" or "Bontsha the Silent," I suspect. Or even better, Roth and Malamud.

They seem to be text messaging each other, fidgeting around, occasionally gazing at their computer screens as if they are taking notes.

I lecture on, pacing back and forth in front of the room, refusing to yield to their distractions.

"Like Adam and Eve, we turn away, at times, disturbed by a sudden gust, a tug of shame. We walk among the trees, hoping that others don't witness the naked truth of our mortality. But this is only half an explanation. Isn't it? Like Adam and Eve, we also desire robust freedom."

Freedom—that's a word the students perk up to. Now they're focused, on the edge of their seats. "Tempted, we yearn for the bright red apple dangling from the knotted and tangled tree of experience," I tell them. "Desiring to be free from the possessive restrictions, those cloying relationships imposed on us, we long for adventure, for independence and self-knowledge. We want to be free."

The students fall back in their chairs.

"What a baby I am," Jeremy said that day. I wanted to embrace him. He wanted his freedom.

"I've only cried twice since this all happened," Jeremy reminds us. "Right after Groff gave me those frightening odds in the emergency ward at Beth Israel, and I thought I might die—and later, that afternoon in the rehab hospital down the Cape, when my friends left."

∼

We are well into September, and during the weekend, Jeremy behaves like an anxious student preparing to return to school after a long vacation. On Monday, he plans to return to his job at the law office for an hour or so. "I'll have to take it gradually," he says, aware that each step of his renewed life demands adjustment now.

On Friday, David set up a makeshift workplace for him downstairs in the old New Bedford office. The creaking stairs slanting up to the second floor of the office, where the lawyers usually practice, are steep and narrow. Jeremy can't negotiate them yet. He won't have a computer downstairs either. The scope of his work will be limited.

When will Jeremy enter a courthouse again? I wonder as I gaze through our living room window. A single sparrow sweeps through the tree-lined valley at the edge of our neighborhood below. Linda's voice floats across the room from the kitchen. She's talking on the phone to a friend about the results of Jeremy's recent immunology test. "They were borderline," she says, her words shifting my attention to her conversation, pushing me to pace, back and forth, over the rugs, across the wooden floor, around the house.

What does Linda mean by "borderline"? The physician said the results were in "the normal range." Granted, on "the low side" of that range, but "normal." I am sure that's what the doctor said. Those are the words he used.

I gaze at the leaves beginning to change their colors on the trees in the valley below. How necessary is it to be precise?—Is it possible?

Saturday night Linda and I drive to Providence to see the play *All The King's Men* at Trinity Rep. The action on the stage jolts me, flinging me back to the first time we traveled to that same theater after Jonathan died, the night they performed *Long Day's Journey into Night*, the O'Neill drama about the ravages of addiction in the family. While that family unraveled slowly on the stage in front of us—their voices like fog horns bellowing in the distance—Linda and I were unhinged as well. We limped from the theater that evening, twelve years ago, our bodies wrapped tight, and silently headed home in the backseat of our friend's station wagon. Near the end of the play tonight, we are shocked again. The son of the lead character, the Governor Willie Stark, suffers a severe injury, a spinal cord trauma. It's as if we're staring into a mirror, watching intently as our own lives flash before us.

The surgeon appears on the stage, talking rapidly to the Governor about his injured son. He tells Stark that his son's spinal cord has been "crushed," his son's future in doubt. I cannot believe what I am hearing. The surgeon's language and description are the same that Dr. Groff used on that terror-laden night almost two months ago, when he talked about our son in Beth Israel. My body trembles while I sit stunned in the audience, the words seeping through my flesh. I am again witnessing the drama of our own son, vibrating on the flat wooden stage in front of me.

Eventually Stark's son dies and so does Stark himself. Jeremy is considerably more fortunate, I know. He will live.

And so will I.

∼

At the end of September, about two months since his operation, Jeremy moves back upstairs at the New Bedford law office. He's closer to the action and seems to be doing well. If you were to observe him from the outside, viewing him from head to toe at a convenient distance, you might conclude he was in remarkably balanced health.

But Jeremy still cannot go into court to try cases, and there are days he pauses on each step as he climbs the steep stairs, slowly contemplating whether or not he will make it to the top. His secretary watches him carefully. She urges him to go home whenever she notices he is struggling to walk—or even to stand.

"I'm glad we have that appointment with Dr. Gomery," he casually tells me for the first time since I arranged the appointment almost two months ago. The appointment is on our calendar for next week.

Jeremy is having trouble measuring success. He can't tell whether he's moving forward or backward. Some days he uses the catheter more than other days. "My blood pressure is up," he tells me one chilly morning after using the monitor I gave him. "The rash is back on my right arm," he says. Is there genuine progress or not?

"You should ask for a new comfortable chair for your desk at work," Linda urges him. "It'll make your back feel better."

But he doesn't.

"Why don't you get a temporary handicap sticker for your car?" I suggest. "Make it easier to park on the street near your office."

But again he is reluctant.

Eventually he drives to the Registry of Motor Vehicles to get a sticker. He stands alone in a slow-moving line. He fights gravity's pull for a long time. Finally, ready to collapse, he secures the required form and marks the appropriate boxes with all the necessary information. He hands the form back to the tired clerk who takes the paper and puts it in a large pile.

They will send him the handicap sticker soon.

∼

In his essay on literature, Tolstoy claimed that a good story was like "an infection"—a slow process penetrating through the skin into the bloodstream. Like an infection, a good story evokes in the reader an unconscious process, unknown and unseen, until the secret of that story finally surfaces. Working through the dark, undetected until that moment of revelation, that secret moves through the reader, haunts him, until it comes to light, Tolstoy suggests. Then, that secret, like an infection, is illuminated. It becomes a revelation.

Literature and infection. Makes sense to me.

I mention this connection to Jeremy.

Jeremy replies: "Well, I'm becoming addicted to reading."

"Oh, I see," I respond. "It's all about infection and addiction."

"Not exactly, Dad," he counters. "But it's like we're always reading a mystery story, although these books I'm reading now are better than most mysteries. There are always hidden clues, secrets to be uncovered, as you move from page to page."

I am impressed by what he is saying.

"Yes, I see what you mean, Jeremy. When one secret is revealed, another one appears, and you want to turn the page and find out what happens next."

"Now you get it, Dad," he says with excitement in his voice. "I see this with the best writers—Coetzee, McEwan. They make you slow down as you read, but they also stir desire."

"Yes," I reply, enthralled by his animation. "Those writers make us want to know what is on the next page, move forward, unravel the mystery as it is created."

"What about Tolstoy's Ivan Ilych?" I continue with a playful smile— "the lawyer who accidentally slipped from a stepladder while fixing his window curtains. Poor Ivan, he was oblivious to the sudden jolt when it happened, unaware of the true condition of his body, until he found himself screaming, flat on his deathbed."

"You've got the wrong story, Dad," Jeremy jokes. "How about Hemingway's Harry—the writer lying on a thin stretcher, dreaming about the stories he hasn't written? Remember him? Poor Harry, lying there at the base of Kilimanjaro, until the mere scratch on his skin inevitably turns to the festering smell of rotting flesh."

Jeremy and I look at each other and laugh out loud.

∽

This time it's Dr. Gomery, the neurourologist.

In the early morning, Jeremy calls to explain his position to me. He's given it considerable thought, mapped out a plan.

"I'll go into Gomery's office first. Then you and Mom can come in after he's examined me and I've had a chance to talk with him. You can ask him your questions then."

"Okay," I tell him. "You're the boss."

What I don't tell him is that I emailed the Omega Institute in New York last night after learning that John of God is scheduled to visit there this coming week. According to their website, there are no more tickets available. But I asked them if John could see Jeremy, perhaps perform some "surgery" on him.

Later, they email me back. John is not allowed to practice "surgery" in New York, they say.

At Massachusetts General, Dr. Gomery proves to be pleasant and likeable; Jeremy is clearly impressed with him. After the doctor examines Jeremy, just the two of them behind closed doors, he invites us all into his cramped office and keeps picking up his phone jokingly: "I'll have to call my bookie in Las Vegas, Jeremy, and place a bet on you. You've made such miraculous progress already. You're a sure winner."

Well dressed with a confident aristocratic presence about him, swarthy and suave, Dr. Gomery exudes good humor and old world charm. Jewish, perhaps from Latin America or Eastern Europe—Mexico or Hungary, I speculate. During our discussion, he refers to "the simple son," hinting at knowledge of the four questions from the Passover texts, and ironically alluding to his supposedly "simple answers" to our complex and endless inquiries. He's subtle and good-naturedly supple. I've seen the type before.

As we talk, Gomery makes clear that most of the information we've gotten about the bladder is just "wrong."

"No one really knows how long it takes for nerves to heal," he insists. "You're getting inaccurate information when people say it'll only take one year." The correct information has been out there a long time, he keeps repeating with a good-hearted tone, but most people, including some doctors, are "stupid" about such matters.

"Nerve regeneration could take up to five years," he says with seasoned authority, while he sits at the side of his desk, his legs crossed, a winning smile on his handsome, aging face.

"Given Jeremy's progress so far, I'm very optimistic about his future. Maybe not 100 percent, but maybe 94 percent recovery. Let's make 2012 our goal.

"Catheterize more often," he tells Jeremy. "Empty the bladder fully each time, every four hours. Make sure your bladder doesn't hold more than 400 milliliters of pee at any time." He's concerned that Jeremy has often carried 1,000 milliliters in his bladder.

Then Gomery surprises us; he's talking about "infection." Like Tolstoy.

"Infection usually has little to do with bacteria from the outside, from hands, for example," he says. "It develops as a threat from the inside, from pee stored too long in the bladder."

"Don't worry about wearing those sterile gloves anymore. Just be sure to wash your hands before and after with soap and water."

Jeremy's body suddenly relaxes with this news. The doctor's words give him comfort. "You know," Gomery says, looking at Jeremy with compassion now, "there're a lot of people self-catheterizing all the time. You just don't know about it. It's not public knowledge."

"What you've had is somewhat like a stroke or heart attack," he continues, as if he were a teacher giving a seminar to attentive students. "The blood supply gets choked off and then the bladder doesn't function properly."

Unlike the other physicians, Gomery tells Jeremy to increase the number of Urecholine pills from three to four and to keep a rigorous record of his urine output for six weeks to establish a baseline. He is giving Jeremy structure and direction.

Before we leave, Jeremy asks Gomery if he can talk to him again alone. Linda and I leave the office, and behind shut doors, Jeremy asks Gomery about his sexual future, about potency and about children. Gomery cannot offer him a definitive answer to these tough questions, but once again with irony and good humor, the doctor has a recommendation: "Jeremy, you need to get a girlfriend and start making a chart."

"I like that guy," Jeremy tells us when we ride home to Dartmouth, comforted by the doctor's easy manner and soothing advice.

∼

On the weekends, Jeremy and I walk around Buttonwood Park, a pastoral retreat I've known since I was a young boy living in the West End of New Bedford. The public park stretches across several acres with green fields and big maple trees, flower gardens and an attractive zoo. It is a difficult walk for Jeremy, his muscles taut, his body nearly breathless at times. But it's a walk we always marvel at, conversing together and sharing visions. We stir energy as we go. Open to the blue heavens, these walks resonate with hope and possibilities, like the voice of William Blake in his expansive mode:

> *And they conversed together in Visionary forms dramatic*
>   *which bright*
> *Redounded from their Tongues in thunderous Majesty,*
>   *in Visions*
> *In new Expanses, Creating exemplars of Memory and of Intellect,*
> *Creating Space, creating Time according to The wonders Divine*
> *Of Human Imagination*

"I'm considering writing a book about all this," I tell Jeremy while we make our adventure through the park on a cool morning in the beginning of October.

"It's easy to walk, until you can't," he replies, as we slow our pace under the maple trees. "You can use that in your book if you want."

That line sounds brilliant to me when I first hear it. Exactly right.

How can those warmed next to the fire understand those who are cold? How can those who are healthy understand those who are ill? How can those who are powerful understand those who are powerless—unless we take the time to listen carefully to each other's stories; unless we risk that border crossing?

And then together we hear the voice of the poet again in the distance, suddenly rushing to us from the horizon:

> *...& every Word and Every Character*
> *Was Human according to the Expansion & Contraction, the*
>   *translucence or*
> *Opakeness of Nervous fibres...*
> *...& they walked*
> *To & fro in Eternity as One Man, reflecting each in each &*
>   *clearly seen*
> *And seeing:...*

It is a careful walk. Jeremy pushing hard, smiling, making progress. Father and son, side by side, the flow of our language stirring the fall air with hope.

Our sauntering done, I wrap my arms around him in the parking lot; he kisses my cheek in return. Then he slips into his car, and behind the wheel, he begins to move away. As he goes, he turns his face toward me and waves through the glass window until he fades from my sight.

Since Jeremy loves the Red Sox, he is focused on the playoff games at Fenway Park. Ordinarily he'd travel up to Fenway to root for the Sox with a bunch of his friends. They are all passionate about baseball and football, chatting endlessly about Manny and Papi, and constantly devising new strategies to win first place in their fantasy leagues.

I hunt around for playoff tickets for him, and finally score two for the first game. Then I realize that on that same Wednesday Jeremy has an appointment with Dr. Groff in the late morning. He cannot travel to Boston, undergo an MRI, meet with Groff and then attend the game in the evening. Too exhausting.

Most people warn me that Jeremy shouldn't go to Fenway anyway. The small and uncomfortable wooden seats in the legendary ballpark, the crowds pushing and shoving along the narrow and cramped aisles, the long walk from Yawkey Way to the box seats—all present unforgiving challenges to Jeremy right now, they claim.

Not ready to accept their advice, I get another set of tickets for the second series, just above the Red Sox dugout, seats that usually evoke instant pleasure—scenes of pastoral peace with the Green Monster in the distance. Jeremy responds with some hesitation: "I'd really rather watch the game on television, Dad. I like that comfortable cushioned chair in my apartment."

"Yes," I agree. "That's probably the best seat in the house anyway."

Fighting his ongoing back pain, Jeremy refuses to yield. He leans on the counter next to the stove in his apartment, cooking jambalaya and chili with his friends, and drinking a few Bud Lites, despite Linda's vigorous objections. His friends encourage him, give him a boost; they want to see him out and about, back to his old self. "Let's get going, Jeremy," they shout.

One Friday, he finally decides to go out after work to Freestones, one of his hangouts in downtown New Bedford. In particular, he wants to meet up with his good friend Chris and say hello to all his other buddies who have been constantly asking for him. Freestones is a gathering place for young professionals, busy and bustling at the end of the work week.

When they see Jeremy back in circulation—his curly hair sparkling in the late afternoon light as he walks through the door—their voices rise with pleasure. "Hey, look who's here," they all yell from the bar, their ties loosened on their necks, suitcoats resting on the bar stools, Guinness drafts in their hands.

His comrades huddle around him. They slap him on his sore back without thinking, and tip their drinks to him with gratitude, celebrating his comeback. Pleased to be in their presence, he pulls himself up, greeting each one in turn. At the crowded bar, Jeremy stays standing and chatting with his friends, his brown eyes opened wide, until he begins to slump. When he leaves to head home, his back is beginning to bend.

∽

Since my advanced literature seminar on the American Transcendentalists meets at the university late Wednesday afternoons, Linda and Jeremy drive to Boston without me on that Wednesday, October 5, the day of the first Red Sox playoff game.

"Well, this is the last time you'll need to see me," Dr. Groff says when they enter his office. He has done what he can for Jeremy. We appreciate his gift, but he has nothing more to offer him.

"Yes, he is a miracle," Groff exclaims, looking at Jeremy straining to hold himself erect in the middle of the examination room. The doctor acknowledges that Jeremy has made a remarkable recovery. "Better than any other patient I have ever had in the grip of such a crisis," the neurosurgeon confirms, accentuating how close to the edge an epidural abscess brings you, what remarkable advances Jeremy has made out of the pit.

"He is a miracle." Yes, these words are rare from Groff, and as Linda explains to me at home later, she could not believe what she was hearing when the doctor made that remark. "I thought that he was delivering that line with some wry and weird humor I couldn't fully understand. I assumed Groff must be kidding."

But Groff wasn't kidding; he was completely serious. For him, Jeremy's ability to walk—his general mobility and developing strength—was indeed miraculous. Jeremy's progress couldn't be explained in any other terms. The doctor had witnessed the disastrous effects of spinal cord injury many times; he knew there was usually nothing to be done.

"A miracle." Groff's judgment adds considerable gravity and weight to our sense of Jeremy's trauma. "Arise, Jeremy, take up your bed and walk." He had said that in Beth Israel, hadn't he?

Dr. Groff has done his best. He promised he would, and he has. We are grateful to the neurosurgeon for his talent and skill. "I'm glad I could play even a small role in your recovery," he said with grace when Jeremy thanked him for all of us before leaving the office that day.

∼

"I'm not going to drink much anymore," Jeremy casually informs me when we again stroll along the paths in Buttonwood Park. It's a beautiful autumn weekend, the leaves burnt-red and yellow on the tall maple trees, the wind whispering gently across the grass. We hear shouts from children on the swings and slides; the ball fields are packed with young athletes; runners in sweatsuits pass us as we go.

We stop, as we always do, at the steps of the Holocaust Memorial at the edge of the park, where we have placed an engraved brick in memory of Jonathan: "Jonathan B. Waxler: Son & Brother," it reads. When I look at it, I wonder why I didn't insist on having Jonathan's middle name spelled out on the brick: "Blake," after the visionary poet.

"I met up with some of my friends downtown after work on Friday," Jeremy explains when we pick up the pace along the path. "I had two Jack Daniels with Diet Coke at the bar, but I forgot my catheter, so I headed home early."

His troubled bladder responded accordingly, measuring about 1,000 milliliters when he first emptied it back at his apartment; he emptied it twice more, each time measuring another 400 milliliters. The bladder didn't settle back down to the normal levels until late in the night. His startled body was warning him.

"I need to drink more water," Jeremy says when we round the corner of the park and head west. "Hydrate the body, work for a pure colorless quality." That's what his friend Dr. Gomery told him.

Finally, in the parking lot, crowded with cars, I watch him slide into his white Volvo. We are finished walking on this wonderful Indian summer day, language bending back and forth between us, at ease, just letting the words flow. Jeremy has his own space, his own time and direction. When he drives by, he nods to me through the car window as he goes.

A few days later, though, he phones early in the morning, his voice jittery, an undertone of panic in the timbre.

"I've got some blood on my catheter, just a spot."

He also reports a slight temperature. "And I feel some small burning sensation when I urinate."

He calls Dr. Gomery in Boston, who gives him an antibiotic, and Dr. Sawyer, who asks him to bring a urine sample over to the local lab.

The antibiotic works quickly, spreading through his bloodstream, and by Monday he is feeling much better; the results of the urine sample indicate the presence of some blood cells, but no sign of infection.

But I am not satisfied. All this volatility seems unfair in the scheme of things. I phone Dr. Anthony Atala, a stem cell expert at Wake Forest in North Carolina and a nationally known urologist. I want more information about this stubborn bladder. His associate, John Smith III, responds, reinforcing, as they all do, the virtue of patience.

"My motto is: 'As the feet go, so goes the bladder,'" Smith says on the phone. He sounds to me like Thoreau, although he is in a science lab, not at Walden Pond.

Smith suggests I read about a procedure on the Internet called InterStim Therapy, which might help Jeremy in the long run. "It's like a pacemaker," he claims. "Electrically stimulates the bladder, usually with good results. It can also help coordinate the sphincter muscles."

Later I google "interstim" on the Internet and find a stray report from a dissatisfied patient complaining about how painful the procedure was.

~

We live inside a cubist painting. Perspectives keep shifting as if there's no solid ground to settle our feet on. Smith sees little reason to use so much Urecholine and thinks Jeremy should cut back. Gomery sees the need to increase the number of pills, as he told Jeremy the last time he was in his office. Smith believes that Jeremy probably is not urinating independently at all yet, just pushing on his bladder to get rid of the excess. Gomery seems to be indicating something more positive and progressive.

And what about all this physical exercise that Jeremy is doing? Perhaps Groff was right. The spinal cord will heal on its own, as much as it can. The nerves will rejuvenate naturally, or not at all. Exercise makes no difference. Recovery is up to the gods.

The addict can only get control of his illness when he recognizes he has no control of it, I once read after Jonathan died. Recovery is up to the gods. Good luck.

Jeremy struggles up the narrow stairs to his law office now as many days in the week as possible. He takes depositions when he can. He works out with the physical therapist at the Faunce Corner Road facility regularly. He goes for muscle massages on schedule. He needs to catheterize every four hours. He is vigilant about possible infections, drinks water, and takes his medication dutifully. He endures chronic back pain and battles pulsating spasms in his legs. No wonder he's drained, especially by the end of the week. Who wouldn't be?

When they tell him at work they have to cut his salary in half because he's not generating enough revenue, he is thrown off guard, shocked and hurt by the blow to his body. He feels it way below the skin—an insult to his integrity and his innate worth. "Don't take it personally," they always say at moments like this. But anyone would take it personally, I believe.

After that blow, Jeremy stumbles in the office. "I think, Dad, I should quit. Look for a new job," he says with a mix of anger and discouragement in his voice. It is unlikely he could get a new job at another law firm, though; not until he is physically stronger, vital again.

∽

I wonder if the French Catholic writer Simone Weil might help me in some of the discussions I am having with my students in the Jewish literature course. In an unexplained way, she reminds me of John of God and the great Jewish prophets.

Weil makes an intriguing distinction between ordinary suffering and genuine affliction. For her, affliction captures the enigma of life itself. It has biblical implications. She quotes King David, Psalm 88, to bring home her point.

> *For my soul is full of troubles, and my life draweth nigh unto the grave;*
> *I am counted with them that go down into the pit; I am as a man that hath no strength:*

King David is not describing ordinary suffering. He is afflicted. God has hidden His face from David, the king who lost two sons and fell to the ground.

David is shaken. Affliction vibrates through bones crumbling to dust. He is terrified, forsaken. He trembles with the trauma of total loss. Uprooted by a ferocious wind, homeless, in ultimate exile, he is lost in the valley of death. The king has come where we all must eventually go. He has arrived at the edge of the lonely grave, the pit.

But yet, there is something more: God will remember David's affliction, and God will revive the Promise He has initiated:

> *Lord remember David, and all his afflictions;*
> *How he sware unto the Lord, and vowed unto the mighty*
>   *God of Jacob;*
> *Surely I will not come into the tabernacle of my house, nor*
>   *go up into my bed;*
> *I will not give sleep to my eyes, or slumber to my eyelids,*
> *Until I find out a place for the Lord, an habitation for the*
>   *mighty God of Jacob.* – Psalms 132:1–5

Yes, David evokes a Vision, the Presence. Suffocating and breathless, he suddenly senses joy springing up from the deep dwelling place of his affliction. How does David achieve such wonder? How does he revive his lost hope? Perhaps it begins through naming, through his poetry and his music. His voice responds to the wound inflicted on him, the wound battering him to the hard ground. The king finds inspiration in the very midst of his agony, and discovers renewed breath in the rupture resulting from his hammering affliction.

"Affliction is an uprooting of life, a more or less attenuated equivalent of death," Weil says. But yet it brings us to a clearing, close to a miracle, near to the mystery that cannot be grasped.

We slip over the border; the fragile body stumbles in excruciating pain; the vulnerable soul is possessed by demons. We cannot speak. And then, having transgressed that border, in the midst of the agonizing terror of that other country, we suddenly glimpse something miraculous. Awe and beauty edge close to us. Affliction itself becomes our neighbor. Rapture brings us home.

"A mother, a wife—if they know that the person they love is in distress—will want to help him; they will at least seek to lessen their distance from him, suffering some equivalent distress," Weil says.

The prophets speak for those without voice for this reason. And we are all prophets. Is it possible?

∼

On a stormy Saturday at the beginning of November, the three of us travel to Boston to celebrate, belatedly, Linda's birthday. There are hurricane winds and rain in the morning, but Jeremy bought the tickets to the musical *Sweeney Todd* a while ago, and the popular show, with all its blood and gore, goes on at the Colonial Theater despite the weather.

Surprisingly, the theater is jammed, and we are swept up by the intensity of the story. The strange, edgy music fills the damp air with intrigue and enthralls us sitting in the semi-darkness. On the stage, the barber wields his sharp razor in his workroom upstairs, slitting throat after throat, silencing his enemies, while the blood drains endlessly from the inert bodies down to the kitchen below, finally to be mixed into the plump pies.

When the curtain drops for intermission, Jeremy slowly moves out into the main aisle to stretch his cramped legs. His bones shake, his body wobbles. A woman, rushing to the lobby, accidently pushes him, and he trips, lurching back toward the seats. Fortunately, he doesn't fall as the woman races forward to her destination at the refreshment stand.

"I told you to bring a cane," I say to him, as we look at each other, stunned with amazement. "When you see them coming, you can stick that cane out like a sword, flash it around and make them back away."

We both laugh at that.

After the show, we weave our way through the heavy rain to our favorite steak house in Boston, Grill 23. The wind still howls, the wipers fiercely slap against the windshield, but we are eager to continue the birthday celebration in the stormy city. Jeremy is tired and uncomfortable, sweating from the damp air. But when the waiter brings our meals, Jeremy savors the large rib-eye steak, juicy and cooked to perfection, and the thin onion rings dripping with his favorite tastes.

He leans back while we chat together about common everyday things. A fortunate family at a finely finished round table, we enjoy ourselves.

"It's been fifteen weeks now," Jeremy reminds us, his broad shoulders resting against the back of his chair. "That's not very long."

Yes, I consider—almost three months, not very long in the grand scheme of things.

∼

With Jeremy for another follow-up visit in Gomery's office, Linda asks the doctor about the InterStim procedure that Smith told me about.

Gomery responds instantly. "Jeremy is way beyond that. There's no need to even think about such a procedure now." The doctor has a knack for making patients feel good and for finding the right words to wrap the body with hope.

"You don't need to keep those military charts anymore," he adds, with all his charm. "And I want you to start a second medication which will increase your urine flow."

It's all standard protocol, but Jeremy and Linda are pleased.

"Most of the nerves haven't had time to regenerate," the doctor claims, "so it is difficult to measure improvement." Whatever natural peeing Jeremy is currently doing is most likely triggered by nerves not directly attacked by the trauma to the spinal cord.

Dr. Gomery wants to generate belief, and he wants to keep me from looking up marginal information on the Internet, as he tells Linda, but when I peer through his optimistic language, I suspect he's simply confirming what everyone else has been saying: "You need to wait." "Be positive." "Have endless patience." Maybe five years from now we can finally calculate the result.

This strategy can only work for so long. Jeremy's aching heart is anxious, Linda's nerves are taut, and I am impatient.

∾

The fragile flesh keeps us alive, skin tightly stretched between the inside and the outside, like a canvas covering over an open grave. The flesh is like language itself, the mediator and manager of signs and meaning. Like the flesh, language attempts to bring the inside and the outside together. What more do we have?

My brother, David, plans a big Bat Mitzvah party at the New Bedford Country Club for Jessica, his fragile but tenacious daughter. Born with severe brain damage, Jessica has bloomed beyond anyone's expectations.

To me her story is our story, too. Despite her massive disabilities, her life has flourished beyond what anyone could have possibly predicted, like a seed that continues to grow and prosper, surprising all of us who care about her. Jessica is a wonder in the thick air, her tall, thin body refusing to be uprooted by a fierce storm. She lives in another country, but she brings us a message from across the border if we listen carefully.

Jessica evokes the anguish of the human heart, vexed and gnarled in the wilderness east of Eden. And Jeremy wanders in that wilderness, too. He walks in the midst of ferocious winds, seeking to regain his dwelling place in the warmth of the noonday sun. At times, he's quiet and subdued, but at other times, he boils with rage just beneath the skin—a storm ready to erupt.

There was just such an eruption a dozen years ago in his apartment near the Boston Common on Beacon Street, soon after Jonathan had died. It was an overcast autumn day, at dusk, and he was alone, lounging quietly in a hard and sturdy oak chair in the middle of the room. Suddenly, for no apparent reason, he raised his hand high in the air and made a tight fist. Then, hesitating just for a second, Jeremy slammed his hand down with a wallop on that hard oak. The impact split the skin and broke the small bones in his hand. He was in a rage.

"How could you possibly do something like that?" Linda asked him later.

"I don't know how it happened," he replied. "I can't believe it myself."

On the Saturday of Jessica's Bat Mitzvah, Jeremy is distraught, torn between loyalties to family and to himself. Jessica's party will be his first exposure since the operation to such a large group of people, a coming-out of sorts. He doesn't want to hide his face from others, but he doesn't want public scrutiny either. He's on edge.

"Should I just go to the synagogue?" he asks. "That's what's most important anyway. Or maybe I should go home after the religious service and rest for a while. Then I will come back later for the dinner at the Country Club.... No, I'll just go to the cocktail party, say hello to a few people, then go home before dinner.... Well, maybe, I should just stay home. Why should I go anyway? I usually don't even go out with my close pals."

When he settles down, the three of us drive over to the ceremony. We sit by ourselves in the crowded synagogue, huddle together and anxiously anticipate Jessica's performance of the crucial Jewish ritual ushering children into adulthood. The Rabbi explains the meaning of each part of the service to the many Gentiles in attendance; the Cantor sings several prayers as the service unfolds. When we are called up to the *bima*, we rise from our seats, mount the stairs to the stage, and gather around the sacred Torah scroll laid out on the table. Then, standing together, the three of us chant the Hebrew blessings for the Torah reading.

Finally, it's time for Jessica. She has studied her passages for many weeks; she is focused and prepared. Approaching the podium, she pulls herself up tall and then looks out over the congregation. Her thin body trembles slightly as she begins to recite her portion. At first, her voice quivers, but her confidence builds and builds, her voice rising now, all eyes on her. Proudly shouting out to all in attendance, she is caught in the moment, resonating with the ritual rhythm of transformation. Vulnerable before the world, Jessica flourishes with verve, glows with satisfaction, as her presence on the raised platform expands and expands, and the hushed congregation, enchanted, reflects back her amazement. When the service ends, we all draw close to her. We are elated, hugging her jubilant body.

A difficult service for Jeremy, he departs the synagogue before the ceremony is finished. He travels home to rest for a while, his nerves pulsating from the rigid seats in the holy sanctuary.

Jeremy reappears later at the cocktail party, dressed in his richly textured blue suit, his neatly ironed white shirt, and his bright red tie. He looks like a distinguished attorney when he enters and gazes across the Country Club packed with guests, many more than attended the synagogue. Charged with the electricity in the air, the guests buzz about Jessica's magnificent performance. She laughs and shouts with a group of her friends in the main room; she is having the time of her life. Orange and pink balloons flash across the walls, green and gold ribbons sparkle from neatly wrapped presents stacked high on the tables, and the deejay spins music amplified by speakers set throughout the club.

Many of the guests are struck by the color in Jeremy's round cheeks, by how well he looks. He stands relaxed at the side of one of the large rooms next to the newly renovated bar, a glass of club soda in his hand. He smiles broadly, encouraging the crowd to draw close, to chat and to wish him good health.

Waitresses circulate through the rooms, hoisting platters brimming with stuffed mushrooms and puffed pastry. With our red wine, Linda and I position ourselves on either side of Jeremy. He is at our center. How few people know about the scar along his spine, I think, the distance he still needs to go.

Jeremy shakes hands with the guests, as they slowly approach him; he talks easily to one after another, lawyers and businesspeople, the old and the young. They are excited to see him, to wish him well. But I know how much remains out of their sight, how much is hidden from view, while they enjoy their appetizers, fine goodies balanced on small paper plates.

What a marvelous occasion, everyone agrees, as they sip their favorite wine from crystal glasses, nod their heads in approval and move on to the next guest they spot from the corner of their eye.

Standing to the side, I am reminded of what the poet W. H. Auden glimpsed when he mused on Breughel's painting of Icarus:

> *In Breughel's Icarus, for instance: how everything turns away*
> *Quite leisurely from the disaster; the ploughman may*
> *Have heard the splash, the forsaken cry,*
> *But for him it was not an important failure; the sun shone*
> *As it had on the white legs disappearing into the green*
> *Water; and the expensive delicate ship that must have seen*
> *Something amazing, a boy falling out of the sky,*
> *Had somewhere to get and sailed calmly on.* – Ovid

~

Linda has her distractions, too. She has insisted on new wooden floors for our house, a new red leather chair for the living room, a new Tempur-Pedic mattress for the bed and new paint for the inside walls. She cleans incessantly, dusts vigorously. "Let's all go to Chicago for Thanksgiving," she suggests. "I'd like to see my cousin Susan and her husband Mickey for a few days." She is determined to fly to the windy city. She is in pain.

The trip seems ambitious to me. Linda argues Chicago might be good for Jeremy. I think it's too much for him. Yet, I'm willing to try anything if it might turn out to benefit Jeremy. Perhaps it will. Maybe the trip will boost his confidence and demonstrate what he can do beyond local boundaries, halfway across the country. How can anyone know for sure?

"We should also help buy Jeremy a house," Linda suggests. Yes, his own house to dwell in. Perhaps that would give him focus like the wind, a roof and door for location.

Chicago proves to be a rough trip, beginning with a difficult and cramped plane ride, followed by an exceptionally long and slow crawl, bumper to bumper, on the freeways during the evening rush hour from the airport out to Evanston, where Susan and Mickey live. The crowds at the airport annoy Jeremy. The stop-and-go traffic along the highway jolts his spine.

"I'm sorry I allowed this to happen," I blurt out when we finally get to the hotel, and I take our suitcases from the trunk of the rental car, lugging the heavy bags to the curb. My tone doesn't seem right, though, sending Jeremy in the opposite direction. We are all frazzled and jumpy, dizzy as we settle in for the night.

It's an uneasy time in Chicago through this long Thanksgiving weekend. Too cold to do much, and not much to do. On Thanksgiving day, we gather around Mickey and Susan's dining room table to enjoy the feast. Susan's free-spirited daughter, Lisa, a schoolteacher who would prefer to be a dancer, has flown in from New York City, and an elderly retired couple, vigorously working on Barack Obama's presidential campaign, join in the festivities.

"The turkey is cooked just right," I say. "Juicy, not at all dry." "Try the cranberry sauce with it," Linda recommends. "And the sweet potato," Susan says. "Don't forget that."

"And save some room for the bread pudding dessert," Mickey chimes in, as we drink a lot of red wine and toast the Democratic Party. "I liked the stuffing best," Jeremy says. He finds peace, resting on the couch most of the afternoon.

The next day we go to the movies to see *No Country for Old Men*, while Jeremy relaxes alone in his hotel room. After the film, we head straight home.

In the end, Chicago proves worthwhile. Although Jeremy has limited stamina, he's able to travel. He's still not sure-footed, but a trip like this one, halfway across the country, gives Jeremy needed confidence amidst such instability and offers some sense of perspective.

No doubt Jeremy is capable of a sustained journey. He's progressing on his pilgrimage. I need to trust him to make his own way.

∽

Jeremy sits on his Barcalounger, watching his big-screen television across the room. He's running a fever. He checked it several times, and it has risen in the last two hours from 99.4 degrees to just over 100 degrees, and now over 101.

On Wednesday, he took two shots in his right arm, one for pneumonia and one for meningitis, injections recommended by his immunologist in Boston. His arm is scarlet and swollen near the entry point. On the phone, he describes pain spreading through his back and arms, and increased redness near the ten-inch scar running up and down near his spine.

Linda and I believe the fever is a reaction to the shots, but it might be something more insidious; we begin phoning his doctors. It's late Friday night, but finally one doctor, on-call, returns our message.

"If his temperature doesn't go down in a couple of hours, you better take him over to the emergency room at the hospital," she says. "It might be a bladder infection."

It's a typical evening in early December; a crisp wind stirs the cold air; shimmering moonlight glimmers on the road as Linda heads over to Jeremy's apartment. An hour later, I come through the door.

"I'm staying here on the couch tonight. Or maybe in the spare bedroom."

Jeremy quickly responds, a flash of anger in his tone: "You ought to leave, Dad. I can take care of myself."

"No, I'm staying," I counter, Jeremy silently pushing against my insistence and struggling for his independence, Linda agreeing with me. Tonight our son needs parental protection, at least until daylight.

Jeremy doesn't argue, just stands there next to the kitchen sink, deadpan, staring at both of us.

"Did you bring anything to sleep in?" Linda finally asks. "I'm going home. You both should get a good night's sleep."

The moon's pale fire guides Linda along the road. Jeremy undresses, changing into his striped pajamas. His eyes scan over his bookcase, choosing a novel by Coetzee to read. Once he settles in bed, I linger at the threshold. "If you feel worse during the night, let me know," I urge him. "If that happens, we might want to take a trip over to the hospital."

Jeremy sleeps in the big king-sized bed, the one we found him lying in when he couldn't move his legs back in July. He has a private bathroom attached to the bedroom and an oversized closet. On one of his dressers sits a television, and near his bed, on a small table, sit several novels in neat piles and a lamp for reading. Jeremy always closes his door when he goes to bed at night and wears ear plugs as if he is trying to shut out the world and finally discover some peace.

I lie on the soft couch in the next room most of the night, listening quietly in the dark to all the sounds of the apartment, the creaking floors, the boiler going on and off. Occasionally, I get up from the couch and walk the few steps across the floor to the bedroom door. I open it just a crack to peek in and make sure Jeremy is sleeping soundly. To me, he looks like an angel.

The following morning, the red blotch is spreading. "It's beginning to hurt a lot, right at the entry point," Jeremy tells us.

Since it's Sunday, Linda and I meet him at the neighborhood walk-in clinic a mile from our house. The staff at the clinic is just switching shifts when we arrive, but a young physician, Dr. Wu, agrees to see us immediately. She prescribes sulfur antibiotics, the strongest oral medication for this type of infection, and she draws a black circle with a magic marker around the red swelling on his arm.

"He's got a bacterial infection under the skin, cellulitus," the doctor claims. "If the swelling expands beyond the boundaries of this circle, then you'll have to take him to the hospital to get antibiotics pumped through the IV."

By Monday, the red spot spills over the boundary line that Wu has drawn, and Jeremy quickly goes with Linda to see his primary care physician, Sawyer, and calls Gardner, his infectious disease doctor in Boston. In my black Toyota Camry, I race to teach my literature classes at the university.

How lucky these freshly scrubbed students are, I think, as I hunt for a spot in the faculty parking lot. How fortunate they are, walking briskly on a college campus, beneath those beautiful pine and holly trees, their electronic notebooks tucked under their arms, their cell phones humming with text messages. They are the digital age; they are electric.

In my Romantic Literature class, I'll ask them what they see in the poetry of Wordsworth, what they read in those lines that describe a "spot of time" inspired by the "beauteous forms" glimpsed in the flow of the river near Tintern Abbey:

> *...Nor less I trust,*
> *To them I may have owed another gift,*
> *Of aspect more sublime; that blessed mood,*
> *In which the burthen of the mystery,*
> *In which the heavy and the weary weight*
> *Of all this intelligible world,*
> *Is lightened...*
> *While with an eye made quiet by the power*
> *Of harmony, and the deep power of joy,*
> *We see into the life of things.*

What is that "blessed mood," that sublime gift which Wordsworth evokes? Do the students sense the "burthen of the mystery" lingering beneath the images flickering on their computer screens? I'd like to know. Do these college students wrestle with their destiny? I bet they do. Does the truth, imageless and deep, tug at them? It must.

"It's not cellulitis," Dr. Sawyer says as he studies the apparent infection on Jeremy's arm. "Probably some kind of allergic reaction to the pneumonia shot. It's as if your body believes it has pneumonia, and your immune system is trying to create antibodies to fight it."

Both Sawyer and Gardner agree: Jeremy has a mysterious immune system. "Don't take any more shots like this."

∼

Linda believes Jeremy should take another trip, a getaway to some warm climate where he can read good books, relax and not worry about the pressure of work or keeping pace with his friend s. He's lucky my brother has given him wide latitude at his law office. They're flexible and want to see him robust and healthy again.

Linda spends hours exploring possible destinations, mainly in Florida. "We should go to a place close to an airport. No reason to sit for long in the car once we get off the plane."

"Yes, I think that's a good idea," Jeremy agrees.

Linda recommends a two-week vacation. The first week she'll stay in Florida with Jeremy, and then, once the college semester ends, around my birthday, December 16, I'll join them for the second week. Not an unreasonable plan, although perhaps it's too ambitious, too extended for Jeremy. Will this kind of trip actually prove helpful? Granted, it's not like the journey to frigid Chicago. Granted, Jeremy needs comfort. But Jeremy also needs his independence, freedom from his parents' watchful eye.

Linda googles Southwest Airlines, checking the schedule carefully. There's a direct flight from Providence to Fort Lauderdale and another one from Providence to Tampa. Fort Lauderdale might be too crowded for Jeremy, we agree, but what can we do in Tampa?

"I like the West Coast," I say, "further down, though, like Marco Island."

"Sorry, but there are no nonstop flights to Marco," Linda responds, sounding for a moment like a travel agent. "And it's too far for Jeremy to travel by car to Marco from the Tampa airport."

"Well, I could make it down the coast," Jeremy chimes in. Linda and I doubt that.

Finally, we decide on an old resort and spa in Safety Harbor, just over the bridge from the Tampa airport. It looks interesting on the Internet and has a rich history, dating back to the beginning of the twentieth century, when people from around the country, including celebrities, came "to take the waters," as they put it in the advertisements on their website.

Sitting on Tampa Bay, with extensive spa facilities, hot tubs, pools, exercise equipment, massages, large public rooms, the resort might work some magic, I begin to believe. Worth a try—it always is—and Jeremy is ready to go.

"The place is wonderful," Linda tells me on the phone as soon as they arrive. "The rooms are spacious, and the balcony overlooks the water."

During the first week, they enjoy exceptional weather, warm with bright sun, temperatures above average for the winter season. They discover a Greek diner that they walk up the street to each morning for breakfast; an ice cream shop close by—with red, white and blue posters on the walls—becomes a destination for their evening stroll. Jeremy spends hours sitting quietly on his balcony, his body absorbing the heat, while he rests, reading good novels. The sun soothes his nerves; the books transport him. Back at home, I finish up the semester, grade the large stack of final papers from students in my classes and fight off the winter cold.

Early Sunday morning, my birthday, heavy snow makes the roads slick, hazardous with ice. I travel to the Providence airport, hoping the plane will leave for the South despite the unsettled weather. On the shuttle from the parking lot, the attendant tells me several flights have been canceled. I check my luggage at the terminal counter and prepare to wait.

The airport bars are jammed. Crowds pack the sitting areas near the Southwest gate. Everyone watches the football game on one screen, the changing flight schedule on another. I am fortunate. My plane to Florida prepares for take off, and before I know it, there they are, Jeremy and Linda, waiting together, and waving, when I arrive at the airport in Tampa.

It's the coldest day in Florida in several weeks, the temperature dropping about twenty degrees since yesterday.

When we get into the rental car, we head for a pastrami sandwich at TooJay's deli: a perfect birthday present, as far as I'm concerned.

The rooms at the Safety Harbor Resort are clean and spacious, just as Linda said, beds comfortable, linens soft, with an old world ambience and charm. I can see Tampa Bay from our window when I look out into the star-lit sky. Exhausted, I sleep soundly in the big bed, dreaming peacefully on the soft mattress throughout the night.

At sunrise, the morning light glistening on the early dew, I gaze through the glass of the patio doors, the view expanding out to the horizon.

Then my body suddenly contracts. I fix on muddy puddles of water stagnant in the marsh between our rooms and the Bay. Couldn't that marsh attract mosquitos and bacteria? And this furniture? Doesn't it have an odd odor, somewhat like the old musty summer camp smell when I was a kid?

We head to breakfast, making our way through the hotel corridors narrow and grim. "Maybe we should move to another section of the resort?"

"Just what we expected," Linda says, looking knowingly at Jeremy.

"Yes, Dad always likes to change rooms at least once," Jeremy responds, shaking his head and laughing as we walk through the exit doors out toward the Greek diner up the road.

We move across the complex to the Towers, a group of newly renovated rooms that offer better views of the bay and stand higher from the ground. This should work well, I think. But as soon as we enter the new room, we run into trouble: Linda spots brown mold growing on one of the pillows on the cushioned chair. "We've got to get another room," even Linda insists. Settled into that other room, in the quiet of night, we hear the air conditioner furiously banging, off and on, without end.

"Yes, that's true everywhere in the Towers," the manager tells us at the front desk the next morning. "It's the way the machinery operates since we worked on the building earlier this year."

"It's all right with me," Jeremy counters. "I wear ear plugs anyway."

By noon, Linda and I journey along the coast up through Clearwater and St. Petersburg, scouting for a fresh place near the beaches. Jeremy leans back on a comfortable lounge chair in the warm sun, reading on his new balcony at the resort, far from the ground. He's glad to be away from both of us for a while. We inspect several places along the coast but can't find anything suitable overlooking the water. Finally, we turn around and head back to Safety Harbor.

Linda and Jeremy begin to relax at the Towers, and by mid-week, I join in their rhythm, easing our way through the Florida breeze. We watch the sea birds circle the sparkling bay. We stroll together over the resort grounds and through the peaceful town. We enjoy the cozy Greek diner and the colorful ice cream shop.

But, as it turns out, one week probably would have been enough in Florida.

∼

"I liked the warm weather," Jeremy announces when we return to Dartmouth. "It quieted the spasms in my legs and made my back feel better."

"Then it was worth the trip," I agree, as Jeremy gives me one of his notable smiles, and we saunter into the New Year, five months from the start of this strange journey demanding patience and waiting.

"It's best when I sleep late," Jeremy says. "That gives me more energy." From now on, he'll try that, too—go into work mid-morning, stay for three hours or so. He has regained his balance and footing in the law office.

"If Winter comes, can Spring be far behind?" the poet Shelley asked.

The New Year

Linda and I fly down to Costa Rica for a week-long vacation at Los Suenos resort on the Pacific side of this Central American country. On sharp, curving roads through the mountains, Los Suenos is about two hours by van from the airport in San Jose.

It's the second week in January, and the first time since the summer we've left Jeremy alone for any length of time. He is happy about all this I am sure, pleased to get some distance between himself and his parents. But I am unsettled as we fly out from Logan in Boston for the long plane ride down to a territory I know little about, a small place without an army, a country bordered by Nicaragua on the north and Panama on the south.

Once we arrive at the resort, I quickly shed the weight of the winter weather up north and swim in the cool water, my skin baking in the tropical sun. I note the large number of young couples around the pool, playing volleyball, laughing and sipping their colorful fruit drinks. Some have young children with them as well.

Our cell phones don't work in Costa Rica, and we've purposely left our laptop computer at home, so we lack easy communication with anyone in Dartmouth. Jeremy has scheduled his first jury trial since his surgery for Tuesday, and he has an appointment with Dr. Gomery in Boston on Friday. I want to be in touch with him.

At the Business Center in the resort, I buy fifteen minutes of computer time and send off a quick email message telling him we're enjoying the vacation. On Tuesday he emails back. "Dad, glad to hear you and Mom are having a good time. I settled the case, so I didn't have to bring it to the jury." He sounds satisfied but tired.

We begin to settle in. Our room offers a breathtaking view opening out to the ocean, and the intricate series of connected pools on the extensive grounds of the resort reminds us of Venice, with bridges and canals mirroring back magic and romance. Yachts bob quietly, up and down, in the cool blue water of the marina. Colorful houses spot the hills. Linda and I swim in the pool and absorb the tropical heat during the day. In the evening, wondering why we don't live like this more often, we feast on finely cooked tuna and drink dry wine.

The natural environment in Costa Rica enchants us as well. We see macaws, a white-faced monkey, crocodiles and a variety of plants and birds as we stroll through the rainforest.

Lounging near the pool one hot afternoon in the middle of the week, I ask a fellow vacationer familiar with the area, "How long is the plane trip from San Jose to Rio?"

My buddy, under his umbrella, orders a drink from one of the many waiters circulating among the guests. "Rio? About six hours," he says, turning his tanned face in my direction.

"I suppose you need a visa and inoculations if you're going into the central regions there in Brazil," I shout over the music blaring from the speakers and think about John of God.

"Yeh, partner, you should have gotten some shots before you came here, too," he responds with little trace of irony at first. "You never know what kind of parasites you'll pick up."

"Did you ever hear of John of God?" I ask him, when the music stops.

"John of God? You're talking to the wrong guy about anyone with a name like that." My new acquaintance spends most of his time in pursuit of pleasure from Costa Rica to Brazil, he tells me. Divorced two years from his wife in Tucson, he works mainly out of Houston now, when he bothers going back to the states.

"Check the bars in Jaco," he suggests as an alternative to John of God. "You'll get a laugh when you see these old American guys walking out of those places with the local girls who look like they're still in high school." And the American college students wandering along the edge of the main drag might give anyone a laugh, too, Linda and I see later when we go into the town; the young Americans proudly carry their surf boards next to their tanned bodies, whether they know how to ride a wave or not.

My buddy at the pool, a consultant he claims, exudes energy, physical and off-center; I puzzle over his self-assured style. "I'll probably head downtown tonight myself," he says, showing his straight, white teeth. He seems to be happy with himself, but he disturbs me. As he chats, the classic tale "Gooseberries" by the great Russian writer, Anton Chekhov, wells up.

In that story, Ivan Ivanovitch, the main character, protests: "We see the people going to market for provisions, eating by day, sleeping by night, talking their silly nonsense…but we do not see and we do not hear those who suffer, and what is terrible in life goes on somewhere behind the scenes."

Ivanovitch is a man behind a door with a hammer. He longs to rupture the comfort of his happy friends who are "at ease only because the unhappy ones bear their burdens in silence." But Ivanovitch doesn't act on his longing. Instead, he joins the silly chatter of his privileged friends.

"I've been rather calm and comfortable," I whisper to myself. But I wonder if I too am being lulled into that territory of blind happiness. Suddenly I wish I could drive up to Mass General with Jeremy on Friday to talk with Dr. Gomery and be at my son's side.

On Friday, Linda and I rent time on a cell phone from a small shop at the marina and call Jeremy to see how his appointment with Gomery went, what the charming doctor told him.

We also make sure Linda's operation for her fallen bladder is set on the calendar in Boston for when we get back. Having postponed that procedure, originally scheduled for last summer, Linda is now prepared to move ahead with it. I understand her need. Even if we can't do anything about Jeremy's bladder, we can do something about hers, we assume. It's not an unusual operation for older women, especially for those who have given birth to children. But yes, I find it strange right now, and I wish she would wait a while longer, until everything else calms down. We've had enough hospital stays for the moment.

When we connect with Jeremy on the cell phone, he reports on his visit to Gomery. He sounds steady, but disappointed: "Dr. Gomery didn't give me any new medicine to stimulate my bladder, and he doesn't want to see me again for six months.

"He said to stop worrying about the bladder. No reason to be anxious. Just wait and everything will work out. It might take a few years."

"It might take a few years." That's the kicker for me, as I stand outside in the plaza at the marina, holding the cell phone to my ear and watching the cool shadows slowly slide across the brick walkway. "It might take a few years."

What better way to draw patients in—get the patient comfortable over time, make what seems extraordinary just ordinary; eventually the patient feels at peace with his condition. "You'd be surprised how many patients self-catheterize out there," Gomery had said when we first met him, hadn't he?

But then I look up from the plaza, over the red bricks, out across the sea waves, rising and falling, out to the edge where the ocean bends back touching the blue sky, out to that edge sparkling now like a crystal mist. And I am home.

Tanned and well rested, the image of good health, Linda and I return from San Jose through Boston to Dartmouth early Monday morning.

Jeremy seems to have done well without us.

∽

I wonder—is there any logical connection between the word "epidural," as in "epidural abscess," and "Epidaurus," the most celebrated healing sanctuary in ancient Greece and the site of a famous ancient theater? Perhaps not, but logic has little to do with sickness and pain and little to do with healing and the arts. There is more than logic at stake in what matters.

John of God at his Casa in Abadiania, Brazil, a spiritual retreat, might very well be similar to those great Greek dramatists, similar to the god Apollo himself, who also worked at Epidaurus. Reading and writing great literature help in the same way John and Apollo help. Reading and writing focus pain in the body and in the text. Similar to the great healers, literature can provide a powerful antidote for the infection polluting our mortal flesh.

An article in a British newspaper reminds me of all this when it quotes the poet Ted Hughes: "The inmost spirit of poetry is at bottom, in every recorded case, the voice of pain—and the physical body, so to speak, of poetry, is the treatment by which the poet tries to reconcile that pain with the world."

To locate pain in a silent world, to articulate it and to give it a shape, perhaps that is our challenge, a particularly difficult challenge because pain often makes the victim squirm and attempts to betray him. Pain rises up to silence human language itself.

Imagine Cincinnatus, one of the most stunning literary characters I have ever encountered. "I have no desires, save the desire to express myself—in defiance of the world's muteness," he says.

In prison, waiting to be beheaded for some unknown reason, Cincinnatus suffers wrenching pain. No one will tell him the date of his execution. Perhaps he will die tomorrow, perhaps next week, maybe next year. In need of support from the prison guards, Cincinnatus stumbles through the long corridors of his confinement: "He plants his feet unsteadily, like a child who has just learned to walk, or as if he is walking on water only to have a sudden doubt...," the novelist Nabokov writes. Cincinnatus is frightened, sick with fright. "But no one shall take me away from myself," he proclaims. He struggles against the silence of the physical world. Refusing to yield, he gives voice to himself. He moves forward through language. Shaping hope, he imagines.

How should we care for those in pain? We cannot stop the pain, kill it. That only numbs us, makes us dead. We must acknowledge the pain. Let it speak.

I witness Jeremy in an unconcealed clearing. His voice flows through the high winds of earth, and he dreams. Seeing a boy falling from the turbulent sky, he is in flight for his freedom. Pay attention.

∽

The second week of the New Year, 2008, Jeremy leans back on a brand new desk chair in his office. He has appeared for several depositions and filed motions in court. He is alive.

His good friends surround him. Like a good book, they stir freedom in him and call desire from despair. There is Mark, the ENT physician for children at Hasbro Hospital in Providence, a loyal pal from Tufts, living with his wife Nicole and their infant daughter in the South End of Boston. Mark comes to stay in Jeremy's spare bedroom when he is on call and needs to be close to the Providence hospital. They watch basketball and horror movies on Jeremy's big-screen television in the living room and enjoy their conversations together, deep into the night. There is Nathan, his old buddy from high school, a lover of venison and hunting. Nathan stops by after work, so they can go out for a beer and discuss women and the future. And Dennis, another devoted comrade from his undergraduate days at Tufts, who lives down the Cape. Dennis checks in regularly. He wants to be sure Jeremy will soon be able to celebrate again every weekend—in Brazil, as they did on New Year's Eve a year ago, or in Chatham, or wherever the wind might take them.

Jeremy's voice carries a smile on its wings. His breath flows before him as if it were a sweet whisper rising gently from the center of his body, a sweet scent beckoning to him. His ears are open to the cadence of the earth, his eyes to the radiance of the arch of the world. In pain, he travels on.

Linda and I meet Jeremy for dinner at The Roasted Pig, a small popular Portuguese restaurant in the North End of New Bedford. He looks well-grounded, although small neuroses begin to creep up in the conversation. "I made a mistake on a court filing," Jeremy says. Nothing of importance, he knows, yet he's worried, masking his concern with a soft chuckle.

Other matters slowly emerge.

"Do you think I take too much Ambien?" he wants to know. "I could get addicted."

"Don't worry," Linda tells him as we wait for our main course. "The dose you're taking is so small; there's no way you could get addicted."

He is talkative, smoothing out his sharp pains and quivering doubts with the flow of language, while we sit around the dinner table, stirring keen joy with scrumptious veal and finely cut potato crisps. It's the first time we've seen him since we returned from our vacation in Costa Rica; his face looks buoyant, his voice sounds strong.

"So what did Gomery have to say?" I ask him about his appointment last Friday, although I already know what the doctor said.

"He really didn't have much to say," Jeremy responds. "Won't have much for a few years."

Jeremy doesn't want to talk about matters of such weight right now; he's delighted with the moment. I change direction and chat instead about local politics, the upcoming weekend, the football playoffs, his fantasy league. Linda wants to know about his plans with his friends. "How's Nathan doing?" she asks. "Any new girls on J-Date?"

At the end of the night, we leave the small parking lot to head home. In the flourish of family conversation, we find renewed promise for the upcoming year.

∼

A couple of years after I graduated from Brown University, I picked up Susan Sontag's *Styles of Radical Will*. I was starting my doctorate degree at the time, working with my mentor, Professsor David Erdman, on my thesis about William Blake. Sontag's book struck me like lightning. It was revolutionary and inspiring, the kind of book you run across once in a great while and always say, I wish I had written that book. It was absolutely brilliant.

Now I am reading Sontag's long essay on the pain of others; I get hooked again when she asserts that we have the right to look at images of suffering only if we can do something to alleviate that suffering, soothe the pain. But I don't think I'm a voyeur when I look at Jeremy. I'm not gazing at a mere image when I look at my son.

Sontag's point is well taken, though. That gaze can become at times lascivious. We can be both fascinated and shamed by what we see. It takes courage not to flinch and look away. But we feel guilty when we do look.

Granted, we cannot gain perspective on the body ripped apart. It has no face, and so we cannot locate an appropriate distance to approach it. That is the body in its death throes, the wounded and scarred body losing its human identity.

In the Beth Israel emergency ward in late July, I was dizzy with abjection, drawn to nausea by the gruesome and horrifying rhythms of the event. I could not find the appropriate distance from my son's body lying flat on the gurney, as if that body were torn apart. I was thrown to the floor then, unhinged.

Suffering is not a mere mistake, not an accident that can be fixed or put aside. It rumbles through the nerves and blood of all of us. I admit that I too have been a tourist on an expensive delicate ship at times, too distracted to notice the wonder of a boy falling out of the sky. But I was mistaken then. Never look away.

The rupture of the body and the battering of the heart, the tearing apart of the soul, they can lead to a transfiguration, an ecstasy in the midst of agony, what the prophets Ezekiel and Isaiah experienced, what St. Sebastian and Teresa of Avila knew. Through the passion borne by sacrifice, prophecy and exaltation arise. That too is worthy of consideration. That is what my son's story teaches me right now as I fly to the sun.

∼

In Providence, Jeremy goes out with a young woman, slightly older than he is. She is one of many, a graphic designer from Warwick, recently divorced with no children. They eat Thai food together in a small restaurant on Benefit Street and talk easily; they chat back and forth across the wooden table covered by a thin linen cloth. Enchanted by the rhythm of the evening, the flow of the conversation, Jeremy plans another date for later in the week.

"I have to prepare, you know," he tells us. "Show up a little early. Go to the bathroom."

He doesn't mention any of this to her.

His body relaxed, his spine erect, he dwells in a place of adjustment. I wonder if he remembers what Dr. Gomery told him behind closed doors in his office the first time they met: "Jeremy, get a girlfriend and keep a chart."

A few days later, when I get home from my office, Linda tells me Jeremy called earlier in the day.

"I had an accident," he told Linda on the phone.

"Are you okay?" she responded, imagining he was talking about a car accident and picturing Jeremy's body jolted by the impact, his back and spinal cord troubled again.

"Yeah, I'm okay now," he replied. "Getting out of my car at the Wareham District Court, I went, all down my pant leg. I jumped right back in the car and called the defense lawyer. Asked him to take care of the motion."

"You mean like what happened walking around Buttonwood Park with Dad last week?" Linda asks, her language guarded.

"Yeh. I had to race home and clean up. Took three showers."

Yes, three showers: one to clean his flesh, one to protect his blood from infection and one to scrub away the unjust insult.

My shoes scuff the tiles; I pace around the kitchen, here and there. These setbacks always set the nerves trembling, twist tight the sinews of the heart. "This will undermine his confidence," I whisper, "make it more difficult for him to return to court; reinforce feelings of public exposure and social humiliation."

At sunset, Jeremy drives over to our house for supper. He's weathered the sudden storm without significant turmoil. "I don't want to discuss it anymore," he says after a few minutes.

He's okay, I see, as he walks across our driveway, his arms and legs gently caressing the air like poetry flowing from flesh shaping language.

We eat roast chicken, asparagus and baked potato around our small glass kitchen table. We discuss a house he might want to purchase in New Bedford, the new girl he is dating, how well he is doing overall. His entire body grins with anticipation. The three of us are flying together through the middle air now. We flourish in clear space, where the wind is light, and the breeze bears us along.

> *For if we go too high, toward the fierce and violent sunlight,*
> *The wax from the wings will dissolve under the heat of the air,*
> *And if we go too low, too closely skimming the waters,*
> *Feathers will lose their lift, weighted by spray and by wave.*
> *Fly between them both, and avoid the turbulence also,*
> *Where the breeze is light, son, let it bear you along.*

∼

A bitter Thursday in late January, the ground is frozen in the silent cold of New England winter. The slate sky hangs silently above the spinning earth. Next week I return to the classroom to start the spring semester. Soon red-breasted robins will sing in the tree-lined valley below, yellow roses will bloom at the edge of our home again, and the freshly cut grass will catch the cool breeze at the break of dawn.

Since the beginning of the new year, Jeremy has progressed steadily, although he's still pushing hard across difficult terrain. His melodious voice resonates with deep timbre, as he moves with the rhythm of friends, the beat of meaningful work, the pulse of the human heart.

We rarely discuss his self-cathetcrizaton, although it remains a thread woven through the tapestry of our conversation. His chronic back pain seems less severe, although he continues with his regimen of medications. He looks lighter, almost free from the draining and insistent reminder of his startling wound.

Jeremy's joy inspires us when we glimpse it on bright and sunny days. When the weather is stormy, and his back aches incessantly, we all share the clouds as we walk together on the earth, dreaming.

Linda and I arrive at Mass General early this Thursday morning so that she can prepare for her bladder surgery, scheduled for 9:45. She has waited a long time for this repair of her bladder, fallen, in part, from the birth of our two sons. Although a reasonably routine procedure, we are both on edge. Linda's body has been riddled with fibromyalgia since Jonathan's death. She rarely does well with pain or anesthesia, and I am particularly sensitive now to any intrusion into the body, especially regarding the bladder.

Linda checks in at the admissions office and then changes into a lightly faded hospital johnny, giving me her clothes in a paper shopping bag. We are brought to a room nearby to wait. Other patients, like Linda, lie on gurneys there, shielded by a half-drawn green curtain; nurses circulate from place to place, gathering basic information, including cell phone numbers for later contact with family members.

At 10:45, an orderly wheels Linda out of the room and down the corridor to the elevator. I walk along at her side, next to the gurney, and then watch the elevator doors open. When the doors close behind her, separating us, I back away. She goes upstairs for her surgery. I go to the waiting area below.

Downstairs, I sit in the family room, while Linda reviews in painful detail her past history with the anesthesiologist upstairs, trying to make clear that she needs a new mix of medicine so she will not get sick after the operation. Then her surgeon arrives, chats with her briefly and reassures her. They are ready to begin.

The family room is crowded, almost every seat occupied, as I wait, reading and pacing, back and forth, checking my cell phone to be sure it's working. Two hours later, the doctor phones from the vestibule of the operating room. "The procedure went without a hitch," he says. "I don't anticipate any problems." Linda should be ready to go home tomorrow after her "shy" bladder, as he calls it, wakes up. I immediately phone Jeremy in his office in New Bedford and give him the good news.

Late in the afternoon, they bring Linda up from the recovery room. Then another patient appears. She seems to be in her fifties, from the town of Beverly, north of Boston. She fell down on the floor in her house, breaking her hip. She looks like a ghost.

Once the new patient is settled, doctors hover at her bedside, talking quietly with her. We cannot help but learn, as she does, that her bones have become very fragile, brittle.

They are sorry, so sorry, but the woman has cancer. The disease has spread extensively through her body, the malignancy showing up now as dark spots on her x-rays. The team of physicians update her condition, off and on, behind drawn curtains, at her bedside, as dusk approaches.

Finally, after a number of bladder scans, around suppertime, the doctors agree to let Linda leave the hospital, and we travel home over that same highway we know so well, from Boston to Dartmouth. The beams from the car lights splash silently on the dark road. The pale fire from the moon guides our way.

It will take several months and another operation before Linda begins to recover from this procedure. Much longer, in fact, than we anticipate. All unexpected. Surprising.

But I think about the woman next to Linda in the hospital room. And I think about Pete, Jeremy's old roommate at the Cape Cod Rehab

Center back in July. And Jonathan. Especially Jonathan. How is he doing now? I wonder. The living and the dead. How will they all do, as time flows on?

∼

On the evening of Jeremy's birthday, almost one year to the day before that startling week that left us spellbound in late July, the three of us return to the Venus de Milo restaurant in Swansea. We celebrate our traditional ritual, feasting on overstuffed lobsters and reviewing the year. It has been a hot summer, but the air is clear and cool tonight, and Jeremy is pleased with his progress. He has a busy week ahead of him: "I'm going to have dinner with my good friend Mark tomorrow after he finishes up at the hospital," Jeremy tells us. "And after work on Thursday, I'm going to that party on the island in Boston Harbor for Nicole's new book. I'll probably stay over in the city."

A few days later, I walk with Jeremy around Buttonwood Park. The maple trees are full, the garden flowers blush with color, and the freshly mowed grass smells sweet from the soft green fields. "I've played a couple of rounds of golf, you know," Jeremy tells me as we move up the path. "And I've made a list for the upgrades for the condo." He has decided to purchase a new place down near the water in Dartmouth. "I'm peeing more often too," he says, although he still uses the catheter regularly.

"So how would you rate your recovery so far?" I ask him as we make the turn. "Give me a rough percentage."

"Oh, I don't know—eighty percent—who knows?" he responds as we approach his car in the crowded parking lot, his light brown eyes sparkling in the summer sunlight.

It is a miracle, truly a miracle, I think, as he slowly drives forward, happily waving and nodding to me as he makes his way home.

I climb the wooden stairs and walk across the balcony to my study. I sit at my table. On that blue pearl granite, I place a sonnet by Rilke, printed out from my Apple computer. I look out across the room to the crafted shelves lining three walls, shelves overflowing with books and journals. I carefully fasten my glasses—wire-rimmed and professorial—around my ears and look down. The sun sparkles through the window as I begin to enter the poem:

> *Be ahead of all parting, as though it already were*
> *Behind you, like the winter that has just gone by.*
> *For among these winters there is one so endlessly winter*
> *That only by wintering through it will your heart survive.* – Rilke

Surely I'll discuss this poem with my literature class this fall, I think, wondering where the time has gone. One day I will retire from the university, but certainly not this coming year—or the next.

I will be in the classroom, talking about literature with my students, when the semester begins. Jeremy will be in the courts, arguing for justice. I shape my life, Jeremy shapes his, as we move through the difficult world, ready to do battle, side by side. The heart survives.

And then I see Jeremy with a smile.
His and mine and Linda's.
And we walk together through that deep valley and over those high plains, the three of us listening to each other with care. We are open to the world now, sauntering through the air, with beds on our backs. The breeze is light; it bears us along. I notice the gaze upon the hill, the sunny one, as we go, pushing on together toward the horizon, grasped by that which cannot be grasped, at such great distance, so fully manifest.

Jeremy Waxler. Earth walker and dreamer. Always and forever, our wonderful son.

About the Author

Robert P. Waxler graduated with a B.A. from Brown University, an M.A. from Boston College, and a Ph.D. from Stony Brook College SUNY. He is currently an English professor at the University of Massachusetts Dartmouth, where he has served as Chairman of the English Department, Associate Dean of the College of Arts and Sciences, and Dean of Continuing Education and Summer Programs.

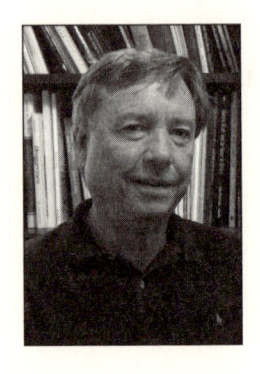

Dr. Waxler is cofounder of the Center for Jewish Culture at UMass Dartmouth, and served as the Center's co-director for fifteen years. He also cofounded "Changing Lives Through Literature" (CLTL), an internationally celebrated alternative sentencing program for criminal offenders.

Professor Waxler is co-author of *Finding a Voice* (University of Michigan Press) and *Losing Jonathan* (Spinner Publications), and co-editor of *Changing Lives Through Literature* (Notre Dame Press). He has published articles in *The Boston Globe*, *Journal of Popular Culture*, *Publications of the Modern Language Association*, *Modern Language Studies*, *Brown Magazine*, and *Journal of Business Communications*. He has written essays for *A Mensch Among Men* (Crossing Press), *The Book Club Book* (Chicago Review Press), *Total Quality Management* (Dryden Press), and *Success Stories* (U.S. Department of Education). The author and his work have been featured in *Parade Magazine*, *Le Nouvel Observateur*, *The New York Times*, and on National Public Radio.

Robert Waxler can be contacted at rwaxler@umassd.edu